Test Yourself Revision

MCQs in
Cardiothoracic Surgery

D1394187

Arjuna Weerasinghe

M.B.B.S.   M.R.C.P. (U.K.)
F.R.C.S. (Eng.)
F.R.C.S. (C-Th)   Ph.D. (Lond.)

St. Bartholomew's Hospital and
The University of London
U.K.

Order this book online at www.trafford.com/07-2621
or email orders@trafford.com

Most Trafford titles are also available at major online book retailers.

Note for Librarians: A cataloguing record for this book is available from Library
and Archives Canada at www.collectionscanada.ca/amicus/index-e.html

Printed in Victoria, BC, Canada.

ISBN: 978-1-4251-5814-9

*We at Trafford believe that it is the responsibility of us all, as both individuals
and corporations, to make choices that are environmentally and socially sound.
You, in turn, are supporting this responsible conduct each time you purchase a
Trafford book, or make use of our publishing services. To find out how you are
helping, please visit www.trafford.com/responsiblepublishing.html*

*Our mission is to efficiently provide the world's finest, most comprehensive
book publishing service, enabling every author to experience success.
To find out how to publish your book, your way, and have it available
worldwide, visit us online at www.trafford.com/10510*

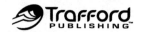

www.trafford.com

North America & international
toll-free: 1 888 232 4444 (USA & Canada)
phone: 250 383 6864 ♦ fax: 250 383 6804
email: info@trafford.com

The United Kingdom & Europe
phone: +44 (0)1865 722 113 ♦ local rate: 0845 230 9601
facsimile: +44 (0)1865 722 868 ♦ email: info.uk@trafford.com

10 9 8 7 6 5 4 3

Note to the Reader

Dedication

To Professor Kenneth M. Taylor, Professor of Cardiothoracic Surgery, Hammersmith Hospital, London, U.K. for over a decade of unstinting guidance and support during my training to be a Cardiothoracic Surgeon and an Academic.

Contents

Preface

Cardiothoracic surgery as a speciality has evolved over a number of decades. In recent times there has been what appears to be a somewhat of a slowing of this evolutionary process. At a time such as this it is important to stimulate trainees in the speciality and provide support.

This book is designed to help provide an opportunity for both surgical trainees as well as others in complimentary specialities and professions to revise relevant topics in the form of MCQs. The MCQ format has been used as in the author's opinion they allow the assimilation of more information per question than would a Single Best Answer (SBA) type of format. There is a section each on Basic Sciences related topics as well as a chapter each on more clinical Cardiac Surgery and on Thoracic Surgery. Each question is followed by five responses and the answers. There follows a paragraph below this that is intended to further learning on the topic pertaining to the question.

The final two chapters illustrate two other question formats – the SBA and the Extended Matching Items (EMI). These questions are followed by the answers. Readers are encouraged to research these topics themselves as an exercise in searching the medical literature.

I hope the book stimulates further study of cardiothoracic surgery and helps trainees preparing for examinations such as the F.R.C.S. (C-Th) and Board Certification.

Arjuna Weerasinghe

Acknowledgements

The author wishes to thank Mr. Alex Shipolini, Mr. Stephen Edmondson and Mr. Alan Wood, all Consultant Cardiothoracic Surgeons at St. Bartholomew's Hospital, London, for their review of the chapters on Basic Sciences, Cardiac Surgery and Thoracic Surgery respectively. My gratitude also goes out to Mr. John Cross of St. Bartholomew's Hospital for taking the time to proof read the book.

CHAPTER 1

The Basic Sciences

Q1 Which of the following are true regarding the t-test?

    A. It assesses whether the means of two groups are statistically different from each other

    B. The t-test judges the difference between the means relative to the spread or variability of the scores

    C. It is calculated by dividing the difference between the means by the standard error of the difference

    D. It is a non-parametric test

    E. It may be substituted for by the one way analysis of variance (ANOVA)

TTTFT

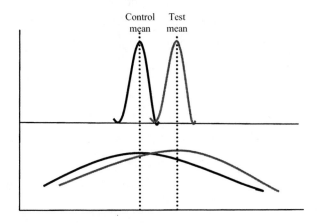

The figure above illustrates how the difference between means can be identical but represent completely different situations with regards the spread of values. The role of the t-test is to incorporate both these facets in the comparison. The t-value will be positive if the first mean is larger than the second and negative if it is smaller. Both the t-test and the ANOVA are parametric tests for the differences between the means.

Q2 Select the correct statements regarding nitric oxide

A. It is synthesized from L-arginine and oxygen by nitric oxide synthase (NOS) enzymes
B. Nitric oxide is generated by macrophages
C. It contributes to post-translational regulation of proteins
D. It protects tissues from reperfusion injury
E. It inhibits the generation of cyclic guanosine monophosphate in smooth muscle cells

T T T F F

It contributes to reperfusion injury when excessive nitric oxide produced during reperfusion (following a period of ischaemia) reacts with superoxide to produce the damaging free radical peroxynitrite. Inhaled nitric oxide (iNO) is a selective pulmonary vasodilator for which the mechanism of action involves guanylyl cyclase activation leading to production of cyclic guanosine monophosphate and subsequent smooth muscle relaxation.

Q3 Which of the following regarding developmental abnormalities of the great vessels of the thorax are correct?

A. In a right sided aortic arch with an aberrant left subclavian artery the left subclavian artery arises as the first branch of the aortic arch

B. A double aortic arch occurs when the caudal part of the right dorsal aorta fails to involute

C. An aberrant right subclavian artery causes the right recurrent laryngeal nerve to originate more inferiorly than usual

D. A pulmonary sling (anomalous left pulmonary artery) passes posterior to the oesophagus

E. In a double superior vena cava (SVC) the right SVC drains to the right atrium and the left SVC to the left atrium

F T F F F

With a right sided aortic arch an aberrant left subclavian artery arises as the fourth branch of the aortic arch. An aberrant right subclavian arises from the descending aorta and passes posterior to the oesophagus allowing the right recurrent laryngeal nerve to pass directly to the larynx. A pulmonary sling arises from the right pulmonary artery and passes between the trachea and oesophagus. Both SVCs drain into the right atrium, the left via the coronary sinus.

Q4 Regarding the oxygen-haemoglobin dissociation curve

A. Haemoglobin is most attracted to oxygen when three of its four polypeptide chains are bound to oxygen

B. Increasing the temperature denatures the bond between oxygen and haemoglobin

C. 2,3-diphosphoglycerate (DPG) decreases the affinity of oxygen for haemoglobin

D. The foetal dissociation curve is shifted to the left relative to the curve for the normal adult
E. Carbon monoxide shifts the curve to the right

T T T T F

The sigmoid shape of the oxygen dissociation curve is a result of the cooperative binding of oxygen to the four polypeptide chains. Cooperative binding is the characteristic of haemoglobin that causes increasing affinity for oxygen as more and more oxygen binds to it. Thus both temperature and 2,3-DPG shift the curve to the right. The leftward shift in the foetus enhances the placental uptake of oxygen, as foetal arterial oxygen tensions are low. Both carbon monoxide and methaemoglobinaemia shift the curve to the left.

Q5 Which of the following are true regarding the thoracic duct?

A. It commences at the level of the second lumbar vertebra
B. In the posterior mediustinum it lies between the descending thoracic aorta and the azygous vein
C. Lymph transport in the thoracic duct is mainly due to the action of breathing
D. It is aberrant in almost 15% of patients
E. Patients who have chylothorax after lung resection rarely require operative repair of the duct

T T T F T

It ascends the posterior mediastinum between the descending thoracic aorta (to its left) and the azygous vein (to its right). Lymph transport in the thoracic duct is mainly due to the action of breathing, aided by the duct's smooth muscle and internal valves. It is aberrant in almost 40% of patients. Chylothorax after lung resection rarely requires operative repair because the leak is usually due to damage to a tributary of the main duct during lymph node dissection. On the contrary chylothorax after oesophagectomy is often high volume resulting from injury to the main thoracic duct.

Q6 Which of the following are true regarding Heparin?

A. It is a carbohydrate that consists of a variably sulphated repeating disaccharide
B. It is a naturally occurring anticoagulant produced by basophils and mast cells
C. It works by inactivating anti-thrombin III
D. It plays an important role in the breakdown of clot
E. It results in the formation of soft clot

T T F F T

Heparin is a member of the glycosaminoglycan family of carbohydrates. It acts as an anticoagulant, preventing the formation of clot and the extension of existing clot. Heparin binds to the enzyme inhibitor antithrombin III resulting in its active site being exposed. The activated form then inactivates thrombin and other proteases involved in blood clotting, such as Factor Xa. Although it is not a thrombolytic, heparin prevents the formation of a stable fibrin clot by inhibiting the activation of the 'fibrin stabilising factor' by thrombin.

Q7 Which of the following are correct regarding surgical needles?

A. The ductility is the resistance of the needle to breakage when subjected to a defined amount of bending
B. The use of a swaged needle increases tissue trauma

C. Reverse cutting needles have an additional cutting edge on the outer convex curvature of the needle
D. In half-curved needles the straight portion of the body follows the curved point
E. Black body surface needles are visualised better

T F T T T

The use of a non-swaged needle increases tissue trauma. The swage is the attachment of the suture material at the non-leading end of the needle to create a continuous unit of suture and needle. Non-swaged needles do not come with the suture attached and the suture needs to be passed through an eye, which may be a closed-eye configuration or split/spring eyed. Due to their extra cutting edge reverse cutting needles are less traumatic to tissue and helpful in the face of tough tissues. In half-curved needles the straight portion of the body does not follow the curved point. Black body surface needles are visualised better due to a relatively 'glare free' surface.

Q8 Which of the following are true regarding drug therapy in transplant recipients?

A. Cyclosporin administration usually is begun immediately postoperatively
B. The major adverse effect of cyclosporine- nephrotoxicity, results from vasoconstriction of the afferent glomerular arterioles
C. Azathioprine is an active drug that inhibits proliferation of T cells and B cells
D. Corticosteroids primarily mediate their effects by interaction with a high-affinity cytoplasmic steroid receptor
E. Mycophenolate mofetil (MMF) is a selective inhibitor of T and B cell proliferation

FTFTT

Azathioprine is a purine analogue converted to active metabolites. These metabolites have inhibitory effects on the proliferation of T cells and B cells. MMF blocks de novo purine biosynthesis. Decreased toxicity of MMF is because T and B lymphocytes use only the de novo pathway in purine biosynthesis, whereas, other cells using both de novo and salvage pathways are not inhibited.

Q9 Quadraple drug therapy for resistant tuberculosis consists of

A. Pyrazinamide
B. Rifampicin
C. Ethambutol
D. Levfloxacin
E. Streptomycin

TFTTT

When resistance is present to the first line drugs rifampicin and isoniazid, quadruple therapy is commenced and continued for at least 18 months.

Q10 Which statements are true regarding the activated clotting time?

A. It is used when heparin levels are too high to allow monitoring with an APTT or when a rapid result is necessary to monitor treatment
B. The ACT has good sensitivity and range with high doses of heparin, but its sensitivity is significantly diminished at lower levels
C. The ACT is measured in international units

D. The ACT may be influenced by a patient's platelet count and platelet function
E. The temperature of the blood may also affect ACT results

T T F T T

The APTT test involves an in-vitro clotting reaction and at high levels of heparin it will not clot. It is measured in seconds.

Q11 Which of the following statements are true regarding cell types encountered in the respiratory tract?

A. Type I pneumocytes are involved in gas exchange
B. Type II pneumocytes comprise 60% of the pneumocyte population
C. Type II pneumocytes are derived from Type I pneumocytes
D. Type II pneumocytes synthesise and secrete surfactant
E. Clara cells secrete surfactant associated proteins

T T F T T

Alveolar type II cells comprise 60% of the pneumocyte population but cover only ≈5% of alveolar surface and proliferate in response to lung injury acting as progenitors for type I cells. Clara cells synthesise, secrete, and recycle surfactant associated proteins.

Q12 Which of the following are true regarding the the Mann-Whitney U test?

A. It is a non-parametric test
B. It assumes that the two distributions are similar in shape

C. It is used for assessing whether the medians of two samples are the same or not
D. It is equivalent to the Wilcoxon rank sum test
E. It does not require independence between samples

T T T T F

The Mann-Whitney test assumes that the samples are random, that there is independence within samples and mutual independence between samples, and also that the measurement scale is at least ordinal.

Q13 Which of the following statements are true about myocardial oxygen consumption?

A. In a steady state, determination of the MVO_2 (rate of myocardial ventilation oxygen consumption) provides an accurate measure of total metabolism
B. Increases in the frequency of depolarisation of the non-contracting heart are accompanied by only small increases in myocardial oxygen consumption
C. Myocardial oxygen consumption is linearly related to heart rate
D. The MVO_2 is increased when a distended beating heart seen soon after coming off bypass, contracts in response to administering Adrenaline
E. Approximately half the MVO_2 in the non-contracting heart is required for those physiological processes not directly associated with contraction

T T T F F

In the failing dilated ventricle treated with an inotropic agent, the increase in contractility reduces left ventricular end-diastolic pressure and volume, leading to a reduction in myocardial tension, which reduces MVO_2. That the total metabolism of the arrested, quiescent heart is only a small fraction of that of the working organ has been known for many years. The small fraction of MVO_2 in the non-contracting heart is required for those physiological processes not directly associated with contraction.

Q14 Regarding the central venous pressure

A. It measures the right atrial pressure
B. It relates directly to the right ventricular afterload
C. In a ventilated patient on PEEP the true CVP is obtained by subtracting the PEEP from the CVP reading
D. During the 'v' wave the tricuspid valve is open
E. Large 'a' waves may occur in tricuspid regurgitation

T F F F F

Subtracting the PEEP from the CVP reading tends to underestimate the actual value. On the other hand excessive PEEP can severely reduce the CVP. Large 'a' waves occur in tricuspid stenosis, pulmonary stenosis and pulmonary hypertension. Cannon 'a' waves occur when the right atrium contracts against a closed tricuspid valve as occurs in complete heart block.

Q15 Which of the following are correct regarding Protein C?

A. It is a major physiological anticoagulant that degrades Factor Va and Factor VIIIa
B. The active form is inactivated by thrombin into the inactive protein C
C. Deficiency is associated with intravascular coagulation

D. When deficient may be associated with skin necrosis on administering warfarin

E. Elevated plasma levels are found in septic shock

T F T T F

Activation of protein C occurs on phospholipid cell surfaces by the action of thrombin, when bound to the endothelial cell proteoglycan, thrombomodulin. Warfarin initially can inhibit protein C more than its inhibition of the vitamin K-dependent coagulation factors (II, VII, IX and X), leading to paradoxical activation of coagulation and necrosis of skin. Activated protein C is used in the treatment of septic shock.

Q16 Which of the following statements regarding the anatomy of the tricuspid valve are correct?

A. The normal tricuspid valve usually has three leaflets and three papillary muscles

B. Congenital apical displacement of the tricuspid valve is called Ebstein's anomaly and typically causes significant tricuspid regurgitation

C. The orifice is smaller than the mitral orifice and is circular

D. The septal leaflet is the largest leaflet

E. The membranous septum and contained A-V conduction system lies beneath the septal leaflet

T T F F T

Ebstein's anomaly is a congenital malformation of the heart characterised by apical displacement of the septal and posterior tricuspid valve leaflets, leading to atrialisation of the right ventricle with a variable degree of malformation and displacement of the anterior leaflet. The orifice is larger than the mitral orifice and is triangular. The anterior leaflet is the largest of the three leaflets.

Q17 The following are true regarding warfarin

A. It enhances vitamine K epoxide reductase
B. It enhances the activity of protein C and protein S
C. It decreases the synthesis of vitamin K dependent clotting factors II, VII, IX and X
D. African americans are relatively resistant to warfarin, while asian americans are more sensitive to its effects
E. Skin necrosis occurs more frequently in women and in patients with pre-existing protein C deficiency

F F F T T

Warfarin inhibits epoxide reductase diminishing available vitamin K and Vitamin K hydroquinone, which inhibits the carboxylation of the coagulation factors at glutamic acid residues, making them incapable of binding to the endothelial surface of blood vessels. The coagulation factors are produced, but have decreased functionality due to undercarboxylation. Warfarin activity is determined partially by genetic factors. Skin necrosis is less common in men and in patients with protein S deficiency.

Q18 Which of the following is/are false regarding the right fibrous trigone of the cardiac skeleton?

A. It is also known as the central fibrous body
B. It underlies the right coronary leaflet of the aortic valve
C. It is connected to the membranous septum

12

D. It is connected to the tendon of Todaro within the right atrium
E. It forms a link between the aortic, mitral and tricuspid valves

T F T T T

The right fibrous trigone is the most inferior part of the arch of the fibrous skeleton of the heart underlying the non-coronary (right posterior) leaflet of the aortic valve. Since it is the largest thickening of the 'cardiac skeleton' it is also known as the central fibrous body.

Q19 Which of the following statements are true?

A. Heparin inhibits anti-thrombin III
B. Bivalirudin inhibits the catalytic activity of thrombin
C. Ancrod acts by enzymatically digesting thrombin
D. Warfarin inhibits synthesis of clotting factors II/VII/IX/X
E. Low molecular weight heparin inhibits factor Xa

F T F T T

Heparin enhances anti-thrombin III. Ancrod acts by enzymatically digesting fibrinogen.

Q20 Which of the following statements regarding the human major histocompatibility complex (MHC) antigens are correct?

A. They are located on chromosome 6
B. They are always identical in monocygotic twins
C. The MHC class I antigens are expressed on all cells
D. The MHC class II antigens are expressed on macrophages
E. They are upregulated by interferon-γ

T T F T T

The MHC class I antigens are expressed on all nucleated cells. Upregulation is aimed at enhancing antigen processing and presentation if a threat is detected.

Q21 Which of the following statements regarding statistical methods are correct?

A. A meta-analysis combines the results of several studies that address a set of related research questions
B. Meta-analysis may be biased towards the absence of a significant effect
C. Propensity scoring stratifies patients into homogenous groups with respect to their probability to receive one of two treatments under comparison
D. Cox regression is a method for investigating the effect of several variables upon the time for a specified event happening
E. Randomised control trials allow the inference of association but not causation

T F T T F

A weakness of meta-analysis is the heavy reliance on published studies, which may bias towards the presence of a significant effect, as it is very hard to publish studies that show no significant results. The propensity score is the conditional probability of being assigned to a treatment group given the covariates, and is used to stratify patients into homogenous groups with respect to their probability to receive one of two treatments under comparison. Randomised control trials are considered the gold standard for assessing causality. Randomisation tends to balance both measured and unmeasured variables between control and study groups.

Q22 Which of the following statements regarding the embryology of the heart and great vessels are correct?

A. The ductus arteriosus is derived from the fourth branchial arch artery
B. The distal portion of the aortic arch is derived from the sixth branchial arch artery
C. The right recurrent laryngeal nerve lies in relation to the distal portion of the right sixth branchial arch artery
D. The bracheocephalic artery is derived from the right horn of the aortic sac
E. The left subclavian artery is formed from the left seventh cervical intersegmental artery

F F F T T

The embryo has two dorsal aortae that communicate with an aortic sac via several pairs of branchial arch arteries. The right dorsal aorta largely and the first, second and fifth pairs of arch arteries involute. The third pair of arch arteries forms the common and proximal internal carotid arteries. The left fourth arch artery becomes part of the aortic arch while the right fourth arch artery becomes the root of the right subclavian artery. The left subclavian artery is derived from an intersegmental artery arising from the dorsal aorta. The brachiocephalic trunk arises from the aortic sac. (Refer to The circulatory system in: Moore KL and Persaud TVN. The developing human: clinically orientated embryology, Sixth Edn. WB Saunders Company, 1998 for more detail.)

Q23 The internal mammary/thoracic artery

A. Arises from the first part of the subclavian artery
B. Is crossed posteriorly in its upper third in the majority of people

C. Terminates at the level of the 8th intercostal space
D. Shows intrinsic atherosclerosis in approximately 5% of patients
E. Intrinsically poor flow (non-iatrogenic) is more likely to affect the right more than the left artery

T F F F F

It is crossed anteriorly by the nerve, which passes lateral to medial. The artery terminates at the level of the 6th intercostal space dividing into the superior epigastric and musculophrenic arteries. Intrinsic atherosclerosis of the internal thoracic artery occurs in less than 1% of patients. The most common cause of proximal subclavian artery occlusive lesions is atherosclerosis and the left subclavian artery is the most common aortic arch branch artery affected by atherosclerosis and therefore, the left internal mammary/thoracic artery is affected more often.

Q24 Which of the following regarding streptococci are true?

A. They are gram positive bacteria
B. Streptococci are aerobes
C. They produce DNAase enzymes that contribute to its virulence
D. Endocarditis is primarily caused by group D streptococci
E. Streptococcus viridans is a term for a large group of generally non-pathogenic, commensal bacteria

T F T F T

Streptococci are anaerobes because they obtain energy by fermentation, even when grown in air. Streptococci are classified primarily based on their haemolytic properties into α, β or γ –haemolytic streptococci. S. viridans, a cause of dental abscesses and endocarditis, is an α–haemolytic streptococcus. It is the β-haemolytic group that is sub-divided into Lancefield groups A to T. Streptococcus viridans organisms are most abundant in the mouth and a member of the group, S. mutans, is the causative agent of dental caries whilst others may be involved in other mouth or gum infections. If they are introduced into the blood stream they have the potential of causing endocarditis.

Q25 Select the correct statements regarding thrombolytic agents

  A. Streptokinase is a fibrin-specific thrombolytic agent
  B. They are serine proteases
  C. Recombinant tissue-type plasminogen activator may be re-administered as necessary as it is not allergenic
  D. Streptokinase is the least expensive fibrinolytic agent
  E. They are effective in non-ST elevation MI (NSTEMI)

  F T T T F

Thrombolytic agents are classified as non fibrin-specific (streptokinase, t-PA and u-PA) or fibrin-specific (alteplase, reteplase, and tenecteplase). Current thrombolytic agents are serine proteases that work by converting plasminogen to the fibrinolytic plasmin that lyses clot by breaking down the fibrinogen and fibrin contained within it. Streptokinase, though the least expensive, is highly antigenic. Thrombolytic therapy is not very effective in non-ST elevation MI (NSTEMI) as the ongoing mechanism of ischaemia is more likely related to impairment of microvascular perfusion than an occluded epicardial artery.

Q26 Regarding the pulmonary artery wedge pressure (PAWP)/ pulmonary artery occlusion pressure (PAOP)

  A. It is normally 12-15 mm Hg

B. The height of the pulmonary wave or the pulmonary artery wedge 'a' wave is the most consistent accurate indirect index for sudden changes in actual left ventricular end diastolic pressure
C. A high PEEP may falsely elevate PAWP
D. In a patient operated for aortic stenosis with a gradient of 100 mmHg, the PAPW measured postoperatively on the intensive care unit overestimates the true preload
E. A PAWP in excess of 20 mmHg, can lead to pulmonary congestion and oedema

F T T T T

The PAPW is normally 6-12 mmHg. It has been suggested that subtracting 1/3 of the PEEP value from the wedge pressure gives a more accurate pressure. Conditions associated with a reduced left ventricular compliance can lead to overestimation of PAPW.

Q27 Select the correct statements regarding apoptosis and necrosis

A. The cell membrane retains its integrity in apoptosis whereas it is lost in necrosis
B. Adjacent cells collectively die in both apoptosis and necrosis
C. Lysosomal integrity is lost in both processes
D. Capsase enzymes are central to the process of apoptosis
E. Apoptosis is an energy dependent process

T F F T T

Apoptosis is a controlled cell death that keeps the intracellular content of the dying cell sequestered. The cell shrinks and starts to display intracellular proteins on its surface whilst the chromatin in the nucleus condenses and the DNA is cleaved into small fragments. The plasma membrane then begins to show a bubbled appearance and small membrane bound bodies break off (known as apoptotic bodies), containing nuclear matter and cellular organelles that are usually unaffected. Necrosis is an uncontrolled cell death, characterised by cell swelling, mitochondrial damage with depletion of energy levels, cell membrane lysis and release of intracellular contents.

Q28 Select the correct statements regarding complement activation

A. The alternative pathway is activated by endotoxins
B. The classical pathway is initiated by activation of C1
C. The classical pathway is stimulated by antigen-antibody interactions involving both IgG and IgM antibody
D. Activation of the alternative pathway occurs with cardiopulmonary bypass
E. Protamine administration causes activation via the alternative pathway

F T T T F

The classical pathway is activated by antibody-antigen complexes. Initiation of the alternative pathway relies on the generation of an activated C3 molecule by various mechanisms including proteolysis by enzymes derived from bacteria themselves, by blood clotting enzymes, and by tissue injury. Complement activation occurs during both on-pump and off-pump cardiac surgery but appears to be more so with the use of cardiopulmonary bypass due to contact activation. Thus, the complement response is caused by the use of cardiopulmonary bypass, by surgical procedures and by anaesthesia. Complement activation occurs via the alternative pathway during bypass and then the administration of protamine causes additional activation via the classical pathway.

Q29 Factors precipitating unstable angina include

A. Platelet aggregation
B. Thrombosis
C. Arterial spasm
D. Dissection
E. Infection of plaque

T T T T F

Investigators, who have applied coronary angioscopy for direct visualisation of offending coronary arteries, have observed complications of an atherosclerotic plaque such as fissures, dissections and thrombus formation present in 60-80% of patients with unstable angina whereas in patients with stable angina uncomplicated atheroma was seen. Vasospasm may be due to release of local mediators at the site of unstable atherosclerotic plaque but sometimes occurs in the context of Prinzmetal angina with normal coronaries. Persistent C. pneumoniae infection is common in unstable coronary artery disease and the association between increased C. pneumoniae IgA antibody titres and fibrinogen levels may indicate that chronic infection could be of relevance to disease activity. Nonetheless there is no direct evidence that infection of plaque is aetiological.

Q30 In familial hypercholesterolaemia the following are true

A. When due to the heterozygous form occurs in 1/500 of the population
B. It is caused by an absent or defective LDL receptor
C. It occurs more often in males
D. In children it is associated with aortic regurgitation
E. Patients with the condition having radial artery conduits should be commenced on verapamil to improve conduit patency

T T F F F

Since the genetic defect lies in chromosome 19 no gender difference is present genotypically. Verapamil interacts with statins to cause severe myositis and the combination is best avoided.

Q31 Select the correct statements regarding the respiratory bronchioles

A. They are lined predominantly by cuboidal ciliated epithelial cells
B. They contain Clara cells that secrete a proteinaceous fluid
C. They are kept patent by incomplete cartilaginous rings
D. They contain secretory glands that keep the air moist
E. They contribute to gas exchange

F T F F T

Clara cells (polyhedral shaped, non-ciliated), are the predominant type and become more frequent distally. They are specialised detoxification cells that populate the epithelium from the level of terminal bronchioles to the alveolar ducts. Occasional cuboidal ciliated cells too are present. From the bronchioles onwards the airways no longer contain cartilage or glands.

Q32 Which of the following are true regarding Cyclosporin?

A. It inhibits lymphokine production
B. It suppresses the calcium dependent production of interleukins
C. It stimulates apoptosis
D. It is available both as an oral and as an intravenous preparation
E. Gingival overgrowth occurs in most paediatric heart and heart-lung transplant recipients treated with cyclosporine

T T F T T

Cyclosporin A inhibits the appearance of DNA binding activity of NF-AT, AP-3, and to a lesser extent NF-kappa B, nuclear proteins that appear to be important in the transcriptional activation of the genes for interleukin-2 and its receptor, as well as several other lymphokines. Cyclosporin A prevents mitochondrial cytochrome c release, a potent apoptotic stimulation factor.

Q33 Which of the following are true regarding the phrenic nerves?

A. They arise from the dorsal segments of the 3rd to 5th cervical dorsal rami
B. They cross the second part of the subclavian arteries bilaterally
C. They enter the thorax between the subclavian artery and vein
D. The left phrenic nerve pierces the central tendon to supply the left hemidaiphragm
E. The accessory phrenic nerve joins the main nerve at the root of the neck

F F T F T

The left phrenic nerve crosses the first part of the subclavian artery. The left phrenic nerve pierces the dome of the left hemidiaphragm anterior to the central tendon.

Q34 Myocardial ischaemia

A. Increases the mitochondrial phospholipid cardiolipin
B. Decreases mitochondrial cytochrome c content
C. Is associated with enhanced glycolysis
D. Is associated with decreased NO production

E. Is associated with increased prostacyclin synthesis

F T T F T

Myocardial ischaemia decreases the content of the mitochondrial phospholipid cardiolipin, accompanied by a decrease in cytochrome c content. The ischaemic heart is dependent on glycolysis for ATP generation, and increased glucose utilisation during ischaemia improves survival. Myocardial ischaemia results in the translocation of the glucose transporter proteins GLUT1 and GLUT4 to the sarcolemma and the increased glucose entry via these transporters contributes to enhanced glycolysis during ischaemia. Under physiological conditions, the activity of iNOS is relatively low but increases following myocardial ischaemia, primarily through activation of invading macrophages by cytokines. Production of NO favourably influences contractile and metabolic functions of the infarcted heart. Prostacyclin and thromboxane synthesis are increased in ischaemia.

Q35 Regarding drugs used to treat infections in cardiothoracic practice

A. Flucloxacillin is inactivated by β-lactamases
B. Imipenam has an extensively broad spectrum of action
C. Fucidic acid is affective against penicillinase producing Staph aureus
D. Vancomycin is preferable to Teicoplanin in the presence of postoperative renal failure
E. Invasive aspergillosis is treated with Ketoconazole

F T T F F

Flucloxacillin is not bound by or inactivated by β-lactamases. Teicoplanin is mainly used in moderate to severe infections with Gram-positive organisms resistant to penicillins. It is not effective against Gram-negative organisms. Alterations in liver and renal function with Teicoplanin are uncommon. Invasive aspergillosis requires treatment with itraconazole or amphotericin B. Recent reports show successful treatment with voriconazole when resistant to the above two drugs.

Q36 Regarding methicillin resistant Staphylococcus aureus

A. Resistance occurs due to the presence of a penicillin binding protein with decreased affinity for the β-lactum ring
B. Outbreaks are equally common in tertiary referral centres and district general hospitals
C. The community acquired strain (CA-MRSA) is a low virulence non-invasive strain
D. It is treated with Vancomycin
E. Alcohol hand washes are an effective sanitiser against it

T F F T T

Outbreaks are more common in tertiary referral centres than in district general hospitals. CA-MRSA has now evolved into a highly virulent and invasive strain.

Q37 The following statements regarding the arterial waveform are true

A. The rate of rise reflects myocardial contractility
B. The area under the pulse pressure curve reflects stroke volume
C. Pulses bigeminus is an indicator of a failing heart
D. Diastolic time relates to myocardial oxygen consumption
E. Pulsus bisferiens is a benign phenomenon

T T F F F

Pulses bigeminus is the result of benign ventricular ectopics. Pulsus bisferiens occurs in HOCM and in combined severe aortic stenosis and regurgitation.

Q38 Regarding the human lymphocyte antigens

A. They are located on chromosme 6
B. HLA antigens typically occur naturally
C. HLA class I gene products combine with $\beta 2$-microglobulin to form functional receptors on most nucleated cells
D. Typing requires live lymphocytes
E. They contribute to both humoral and·cellular immunity

T F T T T

The human leukocyte antigen (HLA) complex on chromosome 6 consists of several highly polymorphic loci. These encode for cell surface proteins important for self-recognition in the immune response. These genes have been classified into major categories. HLA-A, HLA-B and HLA-C encode for Class I molecules. The genes in the HLA-DR, HLA-DQ and HLA-DP regions encode for Class II molecules. These HLA class I and class II alloantigens can induce transplant immunity at both humoral (antibody) and cellular (T lymphocyte) immune levels. The human MHC contains many other Class I and Class II genes (e.g. HLA-G and HLA-DM, respectively) whose products do appear to be as important as transplantation antigens. A third set, the Class III genes, controls a heterogeneous group of proteins that include Complement components C2, C4 and Factor B, Tumour Necrosis Factor, 21-Hydroxylase and Heat Shock Protein-70.

Q39 Which of the following are acute phase proteins that rise in response to tissue injury?

A. C-reactive proteins
B. Albumin
C. Fibrinogen
D. Serum amyloid protein
E. Transferrin

T F T T F

Acute phase proteins are proteins that are produced by the liver and appear in the blood in increased amounts shortly after the onset of infection or tissue damage. They also include haptoglobins, caeruloplasmin, as well as proteolytic enzyme inhibitors such as α-1 anti-chymotrypsin and α-1 anti-trypsin. The stimulus for their production is thought to be inflammatory cytokines such as interleukin-1, interleukin-6 and TNF. Both pre-albumin and albumin as well as transferring levels tend to drop.

Q40 Which of the following statements regarding functional differences between venous conduits and arterial conduits are correct?

A. Veins have a poorly developed internal elastic lamina
B. Heparan sulphate is more expressed in veins than in arteries
C. Production of nitric oxide is lower in veins than in arteries
D. Production of prostacyclin is higher in veins than in arteries
E. Thrombin vasoconstricts saphenous vein whilst dilating internal mammary arteries

T F T F T

Heparan sulphate, a proteoglycan with anticoagulant properties mediated by potentiation of antithrombin III, is less prominent in veins as compared with arteries. Production of nitric oxide and prostacyclin, both potent inhibitors of platelet activation, is lower in veins than in arteries. In saphenous veins, the predominant vasomotor response to thrombin is constriction and contrasts with vasorelaxation that occurs in internal mammary arteries.

Q41 Which of the following are true regarding intimal hyperplasia?

A. It is characterised by the migration of smooth muscle cells into the intima
B. It is characterised by the accumulation of extracellular matrix in the intima
C. It is the major disease process in venous grafts between 1 month and 1 year after implantation
D. It produces significant stenosis of grafts during the first year after implantation
E. It forms atherosclerosis-prone regions

T T T F T

Migration of smooth muscle cells into the intima, with subsequent further proliferation, and subsequent synthesis and deposition of extracellular matrix by activated smooth muscle cells leads to a progressive increase in intimal fibrosis and a reduction in cellularity. During the first year after bypass surgery up to 15% of venous grafts occlude. Between 3% and 12% of saphenous vein grafts occlude within the first month after bypass surgery due to graft thrombosis. Intimal hyperplasia in itself rarely produces significant stenosis.

Q42 The following are correct sources of blood supply to the oesophagus

    A. The superior thyroid arteries
    B. The inferior thyroid arteries
    C. The aorta
    D. The bronchial arteries
    E. The left gastric artery

T T F F T

The cervical oesophagus receives blood from the inferior thyroid arteries. The blood supply to the mid oesophagus is segmental and directly from the aorta. The distal oesophagus is supplied by blood from branches of the left gastric artery.

Q43 Which of the following is false about atrial natriuretic peptide?

    A. It is is secreted in response to atrial distention
    B. It increases renal sodium excretion
    C. It decreases lipolysis
    D. It decreases the glomerular filtration rate
    E. It relaxes vascular smooth muscle in both arterioles and venules

T T F F T

ANP is a polypeptide hormone released by atrial myocytes in response to stress and decreases sodium resorption whilst dilating the afferent glomerular arteriole and constricting the efferent glomerular arteriole thereby increasing the glomerular filtration rate. Increased release of free fatty acids from adipose tissue occurs in response to it.

Q44 The aortic opening in the diaphragm transmits the following

A. The thoracic duct
B. The vagus nerves
C. The phrenic nerves
D. The inferior vena cava
E. The superior epigastric arteries

T F F F F

It is located approximately at the level of the twelfth thoracic vertebra and transmits the aorta and thoracic duct and often the the azygous vein.

Q45 Which of the following are correct regarding the trachea?

A. The adult trachea is 20 cm from the cricoid cartilage to the carina
B. It consisits of 18-22 cartilaginous rings
C. Its mucosa is of a ciliated-columnar type
D. The blood supply to the trachea travels in lateral tissue pedicles
E. The muscular tissue consists of two layers of striated muscle

F T T T F

The adult trachea is 11 cm long at approximately two rings/cm of length. During tracheal mobilisation preserving the lateral blood supply and a tension free anastomosis is paramount to successful outcome. The muscular tissue consists of two layers of non-striated muscle, an outer longitudinal and inner transverse (Trachealis muscle) that forms a thin layer which extends transversely between the ends of the cartilages.

Q46 The following are true regarding Hirudin

A. It is a direct thrombin inhibitor
B. It inhibits factor Xa
C. The ecarin-clotting time is used to monitor hirudin levels
D. It requires antithrombin as a cofactor
E. It is used for the anticoagulation of patients with heparin-induced thrombocytopenia

T F T F T

Hirudin is an anticoagulant peptide that occurs naturally in the salivary glands of the medical leech Hirudo medicinalis and inhibits thrombin. It selectively binds thrombin at each of two sites, the domain that recognizes fibrinogen, and the catalytic domain. Because of the specificity of binding, hirudin does not inhibit other enzymes in the coagulation or fibrinolytic pathways, such as factor IXa, factor Xa, kallikrein, activated protein C, plasmin or tissue-type plasminogen activator. Both the APTT and the ecarin-clotting time have been used to monitor hirudin treatment. In contrast to heparin, hirudin does not require antithrombin as a cofactor. It is FDA-approved for the anticoagulation of patients with heparin-induced thrombocytopenia.

Q47 Regarding the lower oesophageal sphincter

A. It has a normal pressure of 35-50 mmHg
B. Vasoactive intestinal peptide is responsible for maintaining the lower oesophageal sphincter pressure
C. It is normal in the nutcracker oesophagus
D. Relaxation of the LOS is often inadequate or of short duration in diffuse oesophageal spasm
E. It does not relax in acalasia of the cardia

F F T T T

The lower oesophageal sphincter has a normal pressure of 10-30 mmHg. Nitric oxide and vasoactive intestinal peptide are inhibitory neurotransmitters responsible for relaxation of the lower oesophageal sphincter.

Q48 Which of the following are true of the HACEK group of bacilli?

A. They are a group of gram-negative bacilli
B. They constitute the normal oropharyngeal flora
C. They are responsible for upto 10% of cases of infective endocarditis (IE) involving native valves
D. They are the commonest cause of gram-negative endocarditis in people who abuse intravenous drugs
E. They often cause arterial embolisation

T T T F T

The group consists of Haemophilus species (H. parainfluenzae, H. aphrophilus, and H. paraphrophilus), Actinobacillus actinomycetemcomitans, Cardiobacterium hominis, Eikenella corrodens, and Kingella species. They are the commonest cause of gram-negative endocarditis in people who do not abuse intravenous drugs. They have a tendency for large vegetations that cause macro-embolisation.

Q49 Which are true of the papillary muscles and their cordae?

A. The anterior papillary muscle of the right ventricle inserts into anterior and posterior tricuspid valve leaflets

B. The anterior papillary muscle of the left ventricle is larger than the posterior one
C. The mitral valve has basal type chordae only associated with the anterior leaflet
D. Papillary muscle rupture of the mitral valve involves the anterior papillary muscle more often than the posterior
E. Papillary muscle rupture occurs with a relatively small infarction in half the cases

T T F F T

Mitral valve basal chordae are only associated with the posterior leaflet. The posterior papillary muscle is involved in about 75% of cases and the anterior in about 25%. Unlike rupture of the ventricular septum that occurs with large infarcts, papillary muscle rupture occurs with a relatively small infarction in half the cases.

Q50 Differences between the right and left main stem bronchi include

A. The right main stem bronchus is supplied by one bronchial artery
B. The left main stem bronchus is supplied by two bronchial arteries
C. The right bronchial artery arises directly from the aorta
D. The right bronchus is narrower than the left
E. The right main stem bronchus enters its lung lower than the left enters its lung

T T F F F

The right mainstem bronchus is thus more susceptible to devascularisation. The two left bronchial arteries are branches of the proximal descending aorta. The right bronchus (bronchus dexter), is wider, shorter, and more vertical in direction than the left, and about 2.5 cm. long. The right main stem bronchus enters the right lung opposite the fifth thoracic vertebra whilst the left enters the left lung opposite the sixth thoracic vertebra.

Q51 Aprotinin

A. Is a serine protease inhibitor
B. Inhibits plasmin at higher doses than it does kallikrein
C. Inhibits fibrinolysis
D. Inhibits coagulation
E. Decreases postoperative bleeding and transfusion requirements

T F T T T

Aprotinin inhibits several serine proteases, specifically trypsin, chymotrypsin and plasmin at a concentration of about 125,000 IU/ml, and kallikrein at 300,000 IU/ml. Its action on kallikrein leads to the inhibition of the formation of factor XIIa. As a result, both the intrinsic pathway of coagulation and fibrinolysis are inhibited. Its action on plasmin independently slows fibrinolysis.

Q52 Which of the following statements regarding the TNM classification for oesophageal carcinoma are correct?

A. T1 lesions are confined to the mucosal and submucosal layers
B. T2 lesions involve the muscularis propria
C. Regional lymph node metastases are classified as N2 disease
D. In carcinoma of the lower thoracic oesophagus involvement of coeliac lymph nodes is classified as N1 disease
E. In carcinoma of the upper thoracic oesophagus involvement of cervical nodes is classified as M1a disease

T T F F T

While T stage has remained the same over time, N2 disease has been taken out of the system, and M1 has been divided into two subgroups M1a and M1b based on the area affected. Thus regional lymph node metastases are classified as N1 disease. Non-regional lymph node involvement is classified as M1 disease. T3 lesions involve the adventitia and T4 lesions invade adjacent structures directly. The American Joint Committee on Cancer details the classification system.

Q53 Which of the following are true of FDG-PET scanning?

A. A four hour fasting period is recommended before an FDG-PET study
B. ^{18}F used in FDG-PET scanning has a half life of $\approx$110 min.
C. FDG is taken up by tumour cells and hydrolysed
D. The spatial resolution of PET is better than that of CT
E. A negative FDG-PET scan is an indication of a benign lesion

T T F F F

Raised serum glucose decreases cellular FDG uptake because both glucose and FDG compete for the same cell surface receptor. Radionuclides used in PET scanning are typically isotopes with short half lives. FDG is avidly taken up by tumour cells and phosphorylated. The spatial resolution of PET is about 7 mm, much lower than that of other imaging methods, such as CT. A negative FDG-PET scan is not an absolute indication of a benign lesion and carcinoid tumours as well as well-differentiated low grade bronchioalveolar cell carcinoma in the lung may be PET negative.

Q54 Which of the following statements about vasopressin are correct?

A. It elevates systemic blood pressure via vasopressin type 2 receptors
B. Elevated levels are found during heart failure
C. It elevates pulmonary vascular resistance
D. It causes renal dilation
E. It is effective in asystolic cardiac arrest

F T F T T

Vasopressin acts on three different receptors - $V1_a$, $V1_b$ and V2. Vasopressin acts on vasomotor $V1_a$ receptors to elevate systemic blood pressure, $V1_b$ – controls corticotropin secretion from the pituitary and the V2 receptors are renal increasing free water reabsorption. Blood volume and atrial pressures associated with heart failure suggest that vasopressin secretion should be inhibited, but it is not. This is perhaps due to the sympathetic and renin-angiotensin system activation in heart failure overriding the volume and low pressure cardiovascular receptors and causing an increase in secretion. Low-dose infusions cause cerebral, pulmonary and renal dilation (mediated by endothelial release of nitric oxide) while constricting other vascular beds. There is even evidence for the superiority of vasopressin over adrenaline in asystolic cardiac arrest.

Q55 Which of the following are true regarding atherosclerosis?

A. Males are more susceptible than young females
B. An increase in diastolic blood pressure is not a risk factor
C. An elevated plasma homocysteine level is a risk factor
D. LDL oxidation is a main cause of endothelial injury
E. Elevated triglycerides are a risk factor

T F T T T

An increase in diastolic blood pressure is a risk factor. An elevated plasma homocysteine level is recognized as a risk factor for atherosclerotic vascular disease. High plasma levels of very low density lipoprotein (VLDL) are associated with an increased risk of atherosclerosis (triglycerides are a major component of VLDL).

Q56 Which of the following regarding the blood supply to pedicled tissue flaps used in chest wall reconstructions are correct?

A. The blood supply of the rectus abdominis muscle flap is the superior epigastric artery
B. The blood supply of the serratus anterior muscle flap is the lateral thoracic artery
C. The blood supply of the pectoralis major muscle flap is the thoracoacromial artery, when used as a turn over flap
D. The blood supply of the latissimus dorsi muscle flap is the thoracodorsal artery
E. The blood supply of the omental flap is based on either the right or left gastroepiploic arteries

T T F T T

The pectoralis can be used as a turnover flap based on the medial sternal perforators or rotated into the sternal wound based on the thoracoacromial system.

Q57 Which of the following are correct statements regarding the artery of Adamkiewicz?

A. It most commonly arises at T1
B. It most commonly arises on the left side
C. It anastomoses with the anterior (longitudinal) spinal artery

D. It cannot be identified by contrast enhanced CT
E. Injury to the artery can result in devastating ischaemia of the lower spinal cord resulting in the anterior spinal syndrome

F T T F T

The artery of Adamkiewicz is the largest anterior radiculomedullary artery and most commonly arises at T10. The anterior spinal artery may be narrow at the thoracolumbar region and receives a blood supply from the artery of Adamkiewicz, which hence plays an important role in preventing spinal cord ischaemia in the thoracolumbar region.

Q58 Which of the following are correct regarding the Vaughan-Williams classification of anti-dysrythmic drugs?

A. The beta blockers are class I agents
B. Amiodarone is a class III agent
C. Amiodarone also has sodium and calcium-channel blocking actions
D. Many class I compounds also affect potassium channels
E. Calcium channel blockers are class IV anti-dysrhythmic agents

F T T T T

The beta blockers are class II agents. Amiodarone, a Class III anti-dysrhythmic, also has sodium and calcium-channel blocking actions. Many of the Class I compounds also affect potassium channels. With numerous new anti-dysrhythmic drugs and with a much greater yet still incomplete, understanding of drug mechanisms the classification system becomes inadequate, especially for the Class I and III drugs.

Q59 Which of the following regarding Protamine are correct?

A. Protamine sulphate is an acidic protein
B. A large dose of protamine can prolong the whole blood clotting time and activated clotting time via inhibition of thrombin
C. A large dose of protamine can inhibit platelet activation
D. Approximately 1 mg of protamine sulphate neutralises 100 IU of heparin
E. It is ineffective against low molecular weight heparins

F T T T F

Protamine sulphate is a basic protein. It reacts with and neutralises heparin, which is an acid, to form a salt. Postulated inhibitory mechanisms for the anti-platelet effect of protamine include blockade of the fibrinogen binding site of GP-IIb/IIIa, inhibition of platelet factor IV release, and attenuation of platelet response to thrombin, as well as direct inhibition of thrombin. Protamine does antagonise low molecular weight heparins albeit at lower levels of efficiency.

Q60 Regarding acid-base management strategies

A. In the pH-stat method, CO_2 is administered to keep the temperature corrected pH at 7.40
B. The cerebral blood flow is higher at a given temperature with pH-stat management than it is with alpha-stat management
C. In the alpha-stat strategy the pH of the arterial blood decreases with body temperature
D. During rewarming and following bypass, the resulting acidosis is less with pH-stat management than with alpha-stat management
E. Mammals use the pH-stat strategy during hibernation

T T F F T

The alpha-stat hypothesis is about maintaining alpha (degree of ionisation) of the imidazole groups of intracellular proteins constant despite changes in temperature. In the alpha-stat strategy the pH of the arterial blood increases 0.015 pH units for every degree Celsius decrease in body temperature. During rewarming and following bypass, the resulting acidosis is less with with alpha-stat management. With pH-stat management as the CO_2 comes out of solution with rewarming an acidosis results. Mammals use the pH-stat strategy during hibernation whilst reptiles use the alpha-stat strategy.

Q61 Which of the following are true regarding adenosine?

A. It is a potent inflammatory agent
B. It causes conduction block in the AV node via A1 receptors
C. It dilates coronary arteries via A1 receptors
D. Adenosine mediates ischaemic preconditioning via the A1 and A3 adenosine receptors
E. Adenosine induced cardioprotective preconditioning involves opening of K_{ATP} channels

F T F T T

Adenosine is a potent anti-inflammatory agent. It activates four different receptors, the A1, A2A, A2B, and the A3 receptors, all of which are G protein-coupled. The A2a receptor is responsible for regulating myocardial blood flow by vasodilating the coronary arteries. Activation of both A1 and A3 receptors during hypoxia can attenuate myocyte injury.

Q62 Which of the following are correct regarding the moderator band?

A. It is a muscular band extending from the ventricular septum to the base of the posterior papillary muscle
B. It is used to identify the right ventricle on prenatal ultrasound scanning
C. It conveys the right branch of the atrio-ventricular bundle of the conducting system
D. It forms the antero-inferior border between the superior, smooth outflow tract of the ventricle and the trabeculated inflow tract
E. It receives its blood supply from the left anterior descending coronary artery

F T T T T

The moderator band extends from the ventricular septum to the base of the anterior papillary muscle. Haupt and colleagues (Circulation 1983; 67: 1268-72) suggest that collateral flow to the right ventricular myocardium, especially through the moderator band artery, protects against massive infarction in the presence of proximal right coronary artery occlusion.

Q63 Which of the following are true of Complement?

A. It consists of three pathways of activation that converge at component C3
B. The common pathway involves complement proteins C3 to C9
C. The alternative complement pathway is activated by cardiopulmonary bypass
D. The alternative complement pathway is activated in off-pump coronary artery bypass
E. The alternative complement pathway is activated on administration of protamine after weaning off bypass

T F T T F

The three pathways are the classical pathway, the alternative pathway and the lectin pathway. The common pathway involves complement proteins C5 to C9. Coronary surgery with cardiopulmonary bypass, as well as off pump, is associated with a rise in C3a without a concomitant increase of C4a, indicating that it is the alternative complement pathway that is activated. Conversely, the classical complement pathway is activated by the heparin-protamine complex formed after termination of cardiopulmonary bypass, as indicated by an increase of C4a that accompanies the rise in C3a.

Q64 Statins

    A. Slow down the production of cholesterol
    B. Cause liver cells to upregulate expression of the LDL receptor
    C. Are incapable of regressing atheroma
    D. Have no effect on triglyceride levels
    E. Should be taken in the evening

T T F F T

The ASTEROID trial, demonstrated regression of atheroma employing intravascular ultrasound (JAMA 2006;295:1556-65). They do reduce elevated triglyceride levels. It is important that these medications be given in the evening to take advantage of the fact that the body makes more cholesterol at night than during the day.

Q65 Which of the following are true regarding platelets?

A. They are anucleated cells
B. They activate the intrinsic pathway of clotting
C. They activate fibrinolysis
D. Aspirin inhibits platelet cyclo-oxygenase-2 (COX-2)
E. Clopidogrel irreversibly inhibits platelet ADP receptors

T T T F T

The intrinsic pathway of clotting requires calcium ions and phospholipids secreted from platelets. One of the responses of platelets to activation is the presentation of phosphatidylserine and phosphatidylinositol on their surfaces and on the surface of platelet derived microparticles, extruded on platelet activation. Aspirin inhibits the enzyme cyclo-oxygenase-1 (COX-1) that produces thromboxane A-2. The thienopyridines, ticlopidine and clopidogrel block the ADP receptor.

Q66 The following comparisons between the radial artery and the internal mammary/thoracic artery are correct.

A. The diameter of a patient's IMA/ITA is usually greater than that of the radial artery
B. The wall of the radial artery is significantly thicker than that of the IMA/ITA
C. The media shows a dense myocyte architecture in the radial artery, whilst being less tightly organised in the IMA/ITA
D. The radial artery has a monolayered internal elastic lamina, whilst the IMA/ITA has a multilayered one
E. Basal nitric oxide production is better in the radial artery than in the IMA/ITA

F T T T F

The diameter of a patient's radial artery is usually greater than that of the IMA/ITA. It has been shown experimentally that both basal and stimulated nitric oxide production is better in the IMA/ITA than in the radial artery.

Q67 Antithrombin deficiency

A. Is common in neonates
B. Is seen in approximately 2% of patients with arterial thrombosis
C. Occurs as an autosomal recessive trait
D. Is the cause of a low ACT in a patient who has been on a prolonged heparin infusion
E. Is treated with transfusion of fresh frozen plasma

T F F T T

Antithrombin is a late-developing protein with low activities at term, which reach near-normal levels by 6 months of age. Deficiency in antithrombin is seen in approximately 2% of patients with venous thromboembolic disease. Arterial thrombosis is rare. It occurs as an autosomal dominant trait. Antithrombin activity is reduced by long-term heparin therapy and causes heparin resistance on anticoagulating for cardiopulmonary bypass.

Q68 Which of the following basic statistical concepts are correctly described?

A. Data is 'quantitative' if it is in numerical form
B. A cross-sectional study is one that takes place at a single point in time
C. Stratified random sampling may under-represent key subgroups of the population

D. A quasi-experimental design uses randomisation
E. The two-group post-test only randomised design determines whether the two groups are different after the intervention

T T F F T

Generally data is 'quantitative' if it is in numerical form and 'qualitative' if it is not. Stratified random sampling, involves dividing the study population into homogeneous subgroups and then taking a simple random sample from each subgroup. The advantage of stratified sampling over simple random sampling is that it assures not only representation of the overall population, but also of key minority subgroups of the population. The word "quasi" means 'as if' or 'almost', thus a quasi-experiment means almost a true experiment and hence will use matching instead of randomisation. A quasi-experimental design is perfectly acceptable in many situations.

Q69 Which of the following are true regarding the radial artery?

A. It is the larger terminal branch of the brachial artery
B. The superficial branch of the radial nerve is close to the lateral side of the artery
C. It runs between the brachioradialis and pronator teres muscles in the upper forearm
D. It is palpable at the wrist medial to the flexor carpi radialis tendon
E. Radial artery coronary grafts obtained from the distal portion of the artery have a higher vasospastic tendency

F T T F T

The ulnar artery is the larger terminal branch of the brachial artery. The histological architecture of the RA varies along its course, and the muscular component of the media tends to be more developed in the distal portion.

Q70 Which of the following are true regarding the coagulation cascades?

A. The intrinsic pathway is much less significant to haemostasis under normal conditions than is the extrinsic pathway
B. The intrinsic pathway is activated by cardiopulmonary bypass
C. The intrinsic pathway is activated at the time of sternotomy
D. Activated factor X_a is the site at which the intrinsic and extrinsic coagulation cascades converge
E. Thrombin inhibits the coagulation cascade

T T F T T

The intrinsic cascade is initiated when contact is made between blood and exposed negatively charged surfaces such as occurs on exposure to biomaterials in cardiac surgery, hyperlipidaemia, and bacterial infections. The extrinsic pathway is initiated at the site of injury in response to the release of tissue factor (factor III). The activation of factor VIII to factor VIIIa occurs in the presence of minute quantities of thrombin. As the concentration of thrombin increases, factor VIIIa is ultimately cleaved by thrombin and inactivated. This dual action of thrombin, upon factor VIII, acts to limit the extent of tenase complex formation and thus the extent of the intrinsic coagulation cascade.

Q71 Regarding statistical tests that may be used to determine the statistical significance of a 2x2 contingency table, which are true?

A. Both Fisher's Exact Test and the Chi-square test can be used for data in a two by two contingency table

B. For very large tables a large sample approximation may be performed using the Fisher's exact test
C. Fisher's Exact Test can be used when one of the cells in the table has a zero in it
D. The Chi-square value is a good indicator of the strength of association
E. The chi square test is a non-parametric test

T F T F T

Fisher's Exact Test is based on exact probabilities from a specific distribution whilst the Chi-square test relies on a large sample approximation and is more suitable for very large tables. The Chi-square value is not a good indicator of the strength of association, only indicating if an association exists or not.

Q72 Which of the following are correct?

A. The morphological right ventricle is identified by the presence of heavy trabeculations
B. The morphological right ventricle is identified by the presence of multiple chordal attachments to its septal surface
C. The morphological left ventricle is identified by the presence of fine smooth trabeculations
D. The morphological left ventricle is identified by the presence of two papillary muscles on the free walls but not the septum
E. A single left ventricular papillary muscle may be present with left ventricular hypoplasia

T T T T T

A single left ventricular papillary muscle may be present with left ventricular hypoplasia as may occur with a complete AV canal defect.

Q73 Regarding the thoracic sympathetic trunk

  A. The stellate ganglion is formed by the fusion of the first thoracic ganglion with the inferior cervical ganglion
  B. It lies posterolateral to the intercostal nerves and vessels
  C. The first thoracic ganglion is sited inferior to the neck of the first rib between the superior intercostal artery and the ventral ramus of first thoracic nerve
  D. The ganglia of the thoracic sympathetic trunk have both white and gray rami communicantes
  E. Each spinal nerve receives postganglionic sympathetic fibres via a gray ramus

T F F T T

The highest intercostal vein, superior intercostal artery and ventral ramus of the first thoracic nerve lie on its lateral side in that order. Each spinal nerve receives a gray ramus communicans containing unmyelinated postganglionic fibers from the adjacent ganglion of the sympathetic trunk.

Q74 Which of the following is correct regarding reactions to protamine?

  A. A type I reaction is hypotension
  B. A type IIA reaction is an anaphylactic reaction
  C. A type IIB reaction is an anaphylactoid reaction
  D. A type III reaction is catastrophic pulmonary vasoconstriction
  E. Administration of protamine directly into the left side of the heart reduces the cardiovascular effects of protamine administration

T T T T T

A type IIB reaction is an anaphylactoid reaction, and as such being not Ig-E mediated but clinically resembling an anaphylactic reaction. Administration of protamine directly into the left side of the heart via a left atrial line reduces the cardiovascular effects of protamine administration. The reasons that this technique has not found widespread adoption are possibly the infrequent use of left atrial lines and the risk of cerebral air embolism.

Q75 Select the correct statements regarding the vagus nerve

    A. The visceromotor component originates from the dorsal motor nucleus of the vagus
    B. It gives recurrent branches that enter the larynx above the inferior constrictor
    C. It forms the posterior pulmonary plexus posterior to the root of the lung
    D. The right vagus innervates the sinoatrial node
    E. Atropine stimulates the action of the vagus nerve on the heart

T F T T F

It gives recurrent branches that enter the larynx below the inferior constrictor and supply the intrinsic muscles of the larynx except the cricothyroid. The visceromotor or parasympathetic component of the vagus originates from the dorsal motor nucleus of the vagus in the dorsal medulla. Drugs that inhibit the muscarinic cholinergic receptor (anticholinergics) such as atropine inhibit the action of the vagus nerve on the heart.

Q76 Which of the following are correct statements regarding basic statistical concepts?

A. Median is the score in the population that occurs most frequently
B. Variance is the square of the standard deviation
C. The standard deviation of means is called the standard error
D. The dependent variable is the one that the related independent variable is dependent upon
E. The 95% confidence interval tells us that we can be 95% sure that this specified interval contains the true population mean

F T T F T

Mode is the score in the population that occurs most frequently. The median of a population is the point that divides the distribution of scores in half when arranged in ascending or descending order. In the relationship between two causally related variables, the independent variable is the one that is capable of influencing the other, and the dependent variable is the one that is capable of being influenced by the other. The confidence interval quantifies the precision of the mean, and the 95% confidence interval, which is a range of values tells us that we can be 95% sure that this specified interval contains the true population mean.

Q77 Which of the following are correct regarding apoptosis?

A. It is absent in embryonic tissues
B. It occurs following thrombolysis for myocardial infarction
C. It is mediated via both an extrinsic as well as an intrinsic pathway
D. The intrinsic pathway of apoptosis responds to a broad spectrum of both extracellular and intracellular stresses
E. It is decreased in heart failure

F T T T F

Apoptosis occurs in both embryonic tissues during organ modelling and also in postnatal tissues. During ischaemia-reperfusion in humans, up to 30% of cardiac myocytes in the area at risk can undergo apoptosis within the first 16 hours after re-canalisation of the occluded coronary. Apoptosis is mediated via two central pathways, the extrinsic (or death receptor) pathway and the intrinsic (or mitochondrial) pathway. The extrinsic pathway is initiated by the binding of a death ligand to its cell surface receptor, whilst the intrinsic pathway integrates a broad spectrum of extracellular and intracellular stresses. Heart failure involves abnormally elevated but low grade cardiac myocyte apoptosis that persist for prolonged periods.

Q78 Which of the following are true regarding mitochondria?

A. Cytochrome c is located in the mitochondrial matrix
B. The inner mitochondrial membrane contains ATP synthase
C. Most ATP is generated by the proton gradient that develops across the inner mitochondrial membrane
D. Mitochondrial calcium overload is an important factor in ischaemia/reperfusion injury
E. Potassium channel openers protect mitochondria from anoxic injury

F T T T T

In healthy cells ≈15% of cytochrome c is free in the mitochondrial intermembrane space and ≈85% in cristae that are sequestered from the intermembrane space by narrow junctions that can widen to freely communicate with the intermembrane space. ATP is generated as protons are transferred back into the matrix through the ATP synthase complex (chemiosmosis). The cardioprotective mechanism of potassium channel openers includes the direct attenuation of mitochondrial oxidant stress at re-oxygenation.

Q79 Which of the following statements on differences between paediatric and adult hearts are true?

A. The paediatric heart utilises mainly glucose as the oxidative substrate compared to fatty acids in the adult heart
B. The adult heart is better equipped to maintain its adenine nucleotide pool after periods of ischaemia
C. The sarcoplasmic reticulum in the paediatric myocardium is underdeveloped and has a reduced capacity for calcium storage
D. The paediatric heart is more sensitive to catecholamines than the adult heart
E. Paediatric hearts lack well developed pathways of ischaemic preconditioning

T F T F T

A lower level of the enzyme 5'nucleotidase in paediatric hearts is associated with a higher end-ischaemic level of AMP thus preserving its adenine nucleotide pool, and enhancing recovery. The coupling of myocyte β-receptors and adenylate cyclase is less efficient in paediatric hearts and hence milrinone may be better as an inotrope in these patients.

Q80 Which of the following statements are correct regarding the mixed venous saturation (SvO2)?

A. The normal SvO2 is 75%
B. The SvO2 level should be measured from the proximal port of the PA catheter

C. The most common cause of a high SvO2 is sepsis
D. An increase in blood pressure in response to commencing vasopressors will be paralleled by an increase in SvO2
E. Small changes in PvO2 are associated with major changes in the SvO2

T F T F T

The normal SvO2 is 75%, indicating that under normal conditions, tissues extract 25% of the oxygen delivered. In sepsis arterial blood is shunted past the capillaries and into the venous blood causing SvO2 levels to rise. The SvO2 should be measured from the distal tip of the catheter, which lies in the pulmonary artery, thus allowing for adequate mixing of blood. An increase in blood pressure may not always be correlated with an increase in blood flow to the tissues, and therefore it is useful to monitor the SvO2 response concurrently in critical situations. The normal PvO2 and SvO2 lie on the steep portion of the oxyhaemoglobin dissociation curve and thus small changes in PvO2 are associated with major changes in the SvO2.

Q81 Which of the following are correct regarding lung function tests?

A. The FVC (Forced Vital Capacity) is the total volume of air expired after a full inspiration
B. The FEV_1 (Forced Expiratory Volume in 1 second) is reduced in both obstructive and restrictive lung disease
C. Patients with restrictive disorders have a normal FEV1/FVC
D. The diffusing capacity of the lung is decreased in asthma
E. Functional residual capacity (FRC) is measured by spirometry

T T T F F

The reduction in FEV_1 seen in obstructive lung disease is due to increased airway resistance, whilst the reduction in restrictive lung disease reflects the low vital capacity. The diffusing capacity of the lung is decreased in interstitial lung disease and emphysema but is normal in asthma. Functional residual capacity (FRC) cannot be measured by spirometry, and is measured by plethysmography.

Q82 Calcium channel blockers

    A. Bind to L-type calcium channels
    B. Are Class II anti-dysrhythmics
    C. Decrease myocardial oxygen demand
    D. Verapamil enhances atrioventricular conduction
    E. Dilate coronary arteries

T F T F T

They are Class IV anti-dysrhythmics. Calcium channel blockers cause systemic vasodilation, reduced arterial pressure, and thus reduce ventricular after-load (wall stress) and thereby decrease oxygen demand. Verapamil causes atrioventricular nodal block.

Q83 Which of the following are true of thromboelastography (TEG)?

    A. It is a global functional assessment of platelet function, clotting and fibrinolysis
    B. k (kinetic time) indicates how fast clot strength is increasing once clotting starts
    C. A patient being operated as an emergency, having received tirofiban in the cardiac catheterisation laboratory, is likely to show an increase in the MA (maximum amplitude)

D. Aggregometry is a more sensitive indicator of platelet inhibition than TEG

E. When comparing TEG to traditional assays, studies of postoperative bleeding are inherently biased

T T F T T

Tirofiban is a GP IIb/IIIa receptor antagonist and impairs platelet function. Since the MA reflects the maximum strength of the generated clot, which in its turn is predominantly influenced by platelet force generation, it decreases the MA. As TEG summates the contributions of clotting, platelets and fibrinolysis at any one time it is not as specific as aggregometry in isolating the degree of platelet inhibition. In studies comparing TEG with traditional assays an inherent bias towards the TEG arm occurs due to much earlier intervention in the TEG group than in the control group.

Q84 Which of the following statistical statements are true?

A. A type I error occurs if you have rejected the null hypothesis when it is true

B. A type II error occurs if you failed to reject the hypothesis tested when an alternative hypothesis is true

C. β indicates the probability of rejecting the statistical hypothesis tested when in fact, that hypothesis is true

D. α indicates the probability of failing to reject the hypothesis tested when that hypothesis is false and a specific alternative hypothesis is true

E. The power of a test is the probability that the test will reject the hypothesis tested when a specific alternative hypothesis is true

T T F F T

α indicates the probability of rejecting the statistical hypothesis tested when in fact, that hypothesis is true and is the same as a type I error. β indicates the probability of failing to reject the hypothesis tested when that hypothesis is false and a specific alternative hypothesis is true and is the same as a type II error. Power $= 1 - \beta$.

Q85 Which of the following are true regarding the heart and cardiac muscle?

A. The heart can change its force of contraction and stroke volume in response to changes in venous return
B. Myocyte contractile proteins show length-dependent activation
C. The sarcomere is composed of both myosin and actin
D. The troponin complex is made up of two subunits
E. β-adrenergic stimulation decreases intramyocyte calcium levels making the cell hyperexcitable

T T T F F

The relationship between force of contraction and venous return (myocyte stretch) is the Frank-Starling mechanism. Increasing sarcomere length increases troponin C calcium sensitivity, which increases the rate of cross-bridge attachment and detachment, and the tension developed by the muscle fibre. The troponin complex is made up of three subunits: troponin-T, which attaches to tropomyosin, troponin-C, which serves as a binding site for Ca^{++} during excitation-contraction coupling, and troponin-I, which inhibits the myosin binding site on actin. β-adrenergic stimulation increases cAMP which in turn activates protein kinase to increase calcium entry into the cell through L-type calcium channels.

Q86 Which of the following are correct regarding β-blockers?

A. They prevent the binding of norepinephrine/noradrenaline or epinephrine/adrenaline to the β-receptor
B. They are negatively inotropic
C. They are positively lucitropic
D. Labetalol has both α and β blocking activity
E. They cause hypoglycaemia

T T F T T

They are negatively lucitropic. Hypoglycaemia can occur with β-blockers because normally β$_2$-adrenoceptors stimulate hepatic glycogen breakdown and pancreatic release of glucagon.

Q87 Regarding the anatomy and physiology of the oesophagus

A. The oesophagus is approximately 25cm long in adults
B. It is composed of an outer circular layer and an inner longitudinal layer
C. The distal third is composed solely of skeletal muscle
D. The dorsal motor nucleus of the vagus nerve controls the smooth muscle
E. The Meissner plexus carries afferent information to the thoracic sympathetic nerves

T F F T T

It is composed of an outer longitudinal layer and an inner circular layer. The distal third is composed solely of smooth muscle, whilst it is the proximalmost region that is composed solely of skeletal muscle. The dorsal motor nucleus of the vagus nerve controls the smooth muscle whilst the nucleus ambiguus controls skeletal muscle in the proximal portion. The Auerbach, or myenteric, plexus lies between the longitudinal and circular muscle and receives input from vagal preganglionic efferent fibres responsible for smooth muscle control. The Meissner plexus is sub-mucosal and carries afferent information from the oesophagus to the vagal parasympathetic and thoracic sympathetic nerves, and centrally.

Q88 Which of the following are correct statements regarding angiotensin converting enzyme (ACE) inhibitors?

A. They inhibit the conversion of Angiotensin I to angiotensin II
B. They decrease the excretion of sodium in the urine
C. They increase bradykinin levels
D. They should be avoided in women who are likely to become pregnant
E. They should be avoided in diabetic patients having coronary artery bypass grafting

T F T T F

The effects of angiotensin II include vasoconstriction and cardiac hypertrophy. In addition it stimulates the adrenal cortex to release aldosterone, which causes renal retention of sodium and chloride ions and excretion of potassium ions, leading to increased blood volume, and pressure. ACE inhibitors antagonise these effects. A persistent dry cough is an adverse effect believed to be associated with the increases in bradykinin levels produced by ACE inhibitors. The risk of birth defects is present with these drugs. ACE inhibitors reduce the progression of diabetic nephropathy and unless otherwise contraindicated may offer added benefit in these patients.

Q89 Which of the following correctly describe the superior vena cava?

A. It is formed proximally by the union of the right and left brachiocephalic veins at the level of the right first costal cartilage
B. It is joined by the azygous vein at the level of the second costal cartilage
C. The right anterior cardinal vein forms the portion of the superior vena cava that is inferior to its junction with the azygous vein
D. The superior vena caval orifice into the right atrium possesses a valve
E. It is both intrapericardial and extrapericardial

T T F F T

The right anterior cardinal vein forms the portion of the superior vena cava that is superior to the azygous vein and the common cardinal vein forms the section of the superior vena cava inferior to its junction with the azygous vein. The superior vena caval orifice into the right atrium does not possess a valve as does the inferior vena cava.

Q90 Which are correct regarding cardiac electropysiological activity?

A. Purkinje cells are a part of the pacemaker system of the heart
B. Sinoatrial node cells are depolarised primarily by fast Na^+ currents
C. Non-pacemaker cells can change into pacemaker cells
D. The plateau phase in the cardiac myocyte's action potential is due to inward calcium movement through L-type calcium channels
E. Amiodarone increases the effective refractory period of cardiac myocytes

F F T T T

The sinoatrial node is the primary pacemaker site within the heart. Unlike most other cells with action potentials (nerve and muscle cells), the depolarising current is carried primarily by relatively slow, inward Ca^{2+} currents instead of by fast Na^+ currents. Non-pacemaker cells can change into pacemaker cells resulting in ectopic beats and dysrhythmias, for example following a myocardial infarction. Amiodarone is a Class III anti-dysrhythmic drug that blocks potassium channels and retards phase 3 repolarisation, thereby increasing the effective refractory period.

Q91 The azygous vein

A. Is formed by the confluence of the right ascending lumbar vein with the right subcostal vein
B. Drains the bronchial veins from the right lung
C. Drains the hemiazygous veins
D. Develops from the right anterior cardinal vein
E. Terminates at the level of the fourth thoracic vertebra

T T T F T

Developmentally the right posterior cardinal vein in its caudal section becomes a fibrous remnant which remains attached to the inferior vena cava, whilst the rest forms the azygous vein.

Q92 Which of the following are true regarding suture material?

A. Knot strength is related to the coefficient of static friction
B. The more zeroes denoting a suture size, the smaller the suture's diameter

C. Multifilament sutures are more resistant to microorganisms than are monofilament ones
D. The absorptive mechanism is enzymatic degradation for synthetic suture materials
E. PDS is an absorbable polyester monofilament suture made of polydioxanone

T T F F T

The knot strength is the amount of force necessary to cause a knot to slip and is related to the coefficient of static friction and the plasticity of the individual suture material. Because multifilament materials have increased capillarity, the increased absorption of fluid may act as a tract for the introduction of pathogens. The absorptive mechanism is enzymatic degradation for natural suture materials and hydrolysis for synthetic suture materials.

Q93 Which of the following are true of troponin?

A. Troponin is a component of thick filaments
B. Troponin-C serves as a binding site for Ca^{++}
C. Troponin-I inhibits the myosin binding site on actin
D. Troponin-T attaches to tropomyosin
E. Decreased cardiac Troponin-T levels are found in chronic renal failure

F T T T F

Troponin is a component of thin filaments as are actin and tropomyosin. Human cardiac troponin I is present in cardiac tissue as a single isoform with molecular weight 29 kDa, whereas skeletal muscles troponin I is present as two isoforms. Elevated serum concentrations of cardiac troponin-T and, to a lesser degree cardiac troponin-I may be found in patients with chronic renal failure, with or without evidence of overt coronary artery disease, possibly as a result of sub-clinical myocardial damage and/or a prolonged half-life of the marker in the serum.

Q94 Which of the following statements are correct regarding sample size justification and power analysis when designing a study?

A. Maximum power is usually achieved by having equal numbers in the two groups
B. The power of a study is the probability of rejecting the null hypothesis when it is true
C. A larger total sample size is required to maintain a fixed power with a study in which the group sizes are balanced than with an imbalanced one
D. If the sample size were limited by resources, and the significance level fixed in advance, one could arbitrarily increase the power of the study by postulating larger effect sizes
E. With finite populations, corrections are allowed that reduce the sample size slightly

T F F T T

The probability of rejecting the null hypothesis when it is false is termed the power and is defined as $1-\beta$. The probability of a type II error, known as β, occurs if the null hypothesis is in fact false but we fail to reject it. If the allocation ratio is allowed to exceed 2:1 with the same total sample size the power falls rapidly and a considerably larger total sample size is required to maintain a fixed power. When fixing sample size caution is required as often the estimate of the effect of an intervention often proves too optimistic, resulting in many trials which are too small.

Q95 Clara cells of the lower respiratory tract are correctly described as

    A. Non-mucous and non-ciliated secretory cells
    B. Being responsible for detoxifying harmful substances inhaled into the lungs
    C. Containing cytochrome P-450 enzymes
    D. Being mitotically inactive cells.
    E. Synthesising and secreting material lining the bronchiolar lumen

T T T F T

They are responsible for detoxifying harmful substances inhaled into the lungs. Clara cells accomplish this with cytochrome P-450 enzymes found in their smooth endoplasmic reticulum. Clara cells are mitotically active and divide and differentiate to form both ciliated and non-ciliated epithelial cells and secrete proteins such as antibodies and lysosymes.

Q96 Which of the following statements is/are false regarding antigen presentation by the MHCs?

    A. MHC class I antigens are required for the action of CD 8 positive cytotoxic T cells
    B. MHC class II antigens are essential to T helper cells
    C. MHC class I molecules present peptides derived from cytosolic proteins
    D. The MHC class I-dependent pathway of antigen presentation is the primary pathway for a virus-infected cell to signal for help
    E. Class I MHC's play a central role in the presentation of bacteria that might be infecting a sternal wound

T T T T F

The MHC class I molecule's peptide-binding site is in the lumen of the ER. As viruses infect a cell by entering its cytoplasm, this cytosolic, MHC class I-dependent pathway of antigen presentation is the primary way for a virus-infected cell to signal T cells. MHC class I molecules generally interact exclusively with $CD8^+$ ("cytotoxic") T cells. MHC class I presentation is often called the cytosolic or endogenous pathway. The peptides presented by class II molecules are derived from extracellular proteins and not cytosolic as with class I molecules. Thus the MHC class II-dependent pathway of antigen presentation is called the endocytic or exogenous pathway. Loading of class II molecules must still occur inside the cell; extracellular proteins are endocytosed, digested in lysosomes, and bound by the class II MHC molecule prior to the molecule's migration to the plasma membrane. Because class II MHC is loaded with extracellular proteins, it is mainly concerned with presentation of extracellular pathogens such as bacteria in an infected wound.

Q97 Which of the following are correct regarding the elcectrocardiogram (ECG/EKG)?

A. The electrocardiogram is recorded on paper travelling at a rate of 25 mm/s
B. Each small square is 1 mm wide and equivalent to 0.04 s
C. The normal range for the cardiac axis is between $-30°$ and $90°$
D. Sinus node automaticity is represented by the P wave on the surface ECG
E. Prolonged repolarisation results in lengthening of the QT interval

T T T F T

Sinus node automaticity is not recorded on the surface ECG. Activation of the atrial myocardium as a result of sinus node automaticity produces the P wave. The Q-T interval represents the time for electrical activation and inactivation of the ventricles. In the long Q-T syndrome the Q-T interval is prolonged and patients with the condition are susceptible to 'Torsade des pointes'.

Q98 Which of the following correctly describe macrophages?

A. They are the progenitor cell for circulating monocytes
B. They produce plasminogen activator
C. They activate leucocytes by producing interleukin-1
D. They are contained within fatty streaks
E. Foam cell formation, the hallmark of early atherosclerosis, is the result of enhanced cellular uptake of plasma high density lipoprotein into macrophages

F T T T F

Macrophages are derived from circulating monocytes. Fatty streaks, contain macrophage foam cells that are derived from recruited monocytes. Macrophage cholesterol accumulation and foam cell formation, the hallmark of early atherosclerosis, is the result of enhanced cellular uptake of plasma low density lipoprotein, which undergoes oxidative modifications in order to be taken up at an enhanced rate by them.

Q99 The following are correct regarding a standard normal distribution

A. The standard normal distribution is a normal distribution where the mean, the median and the mode are the same
B. It by definition has a standard deviation of 2

C. A normal distribution can be transformed into a standard normal distribution using a formula
D. The standard normal distribution is also called the z distribution
E. The z score reflects the number of standard deviations above or below the mean the value of interest is

F F T T T

The standard normal distribution is a normal distribution with a mean of 0 and a standard deviation of 1. It is used to compare two or more distributions of data or to estimate or to compute probabilities of events involving normal distributions. The z score for an item indicates how far and in what direction, that item deviates from its distribution's mean, expressed in units of its distribution's standard deviation. Thus a z score of 2 indicates two standard deviations above the mean and a z score of -2 indicates two standard deviations below the mean.

Q100 Which of the following statements about inodilator drugs are correct?

A. They are naturally occurring catecholamines that binds to both α- and β-receptors
B. They are characterised by acute tolerance
C. They sensitise troponin C in heart muscle cells to calcium
D. They mediate vasodilation by opening Ca^{2+} channels in vascular smooth muscle
E. They have a high propensity to cause dysrythmias

F F T F F

Dopamine is a naturally occurring catecholamine that binds to both α- and β-receptors. Acute tolerance is not a feature.

Levosimendan is a new inodilator drug that sensitises troponin C in heart muscle cells to calcium, thus improving contractility. It also has a vasodilatory effect, by opening ATP-sensitive potassium channels (K_{ATP}) in vascular smooth muscle to cause smooth muscle relaxation. The Milrinone Multicentre Trial Group compared milrinone with dobutamine and found dobutamine was associated with a significantly higher incidence of new atrial fibrillation.

CHAPTER 2

Cardiac Surgery

Q1 The following figure· depicts the surgeon's view of the tricuspid valve. The three leaflets are named. Which of the following statements are correct?

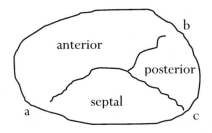

A. A De Vega annuloplasty suture is placed between 'a' and 'b' to reduce the annulus at the base of the anterior leaflet
B. Bicuspidisation is performed for regurgitation by placement of a suture between 'b' and 'c' to obliterate the posterior leaflet
C. A tricuspid annuloplasty ring is an incomplete ring with a gap near the point 'c'
D. Bicuspidisation when performed for stenosis is achieved by commisurotomy at points 'a' and 'b'
E. Closure of a membranous ventricular defect is performed through the tricuspid valve by retracting the leaflets near point 'a'

F T F F T

A De Vega annuloplasty suture is placed from 'a' through 'b' to 'c' such that the annulus at the base of the posterior and anterior leaflets is reduced in size. A tricuspid annuloplasty ring is an incomplete ring with a gap near the point 'a' to avoid damage to the atrio-ventricular conducting tissue. Whilst it is likely that tricuspid stenosis is managed by biological valve replacement, the pathology may be amenable to bicuspidisation by commisurotomy at the antero-septal (a) and postero-septal (c) commisures.

Q2 Which of the following statements regarding mortality for the following procedures are correct?

A. Female gender is associated with a worse operative mortality from coronary artery bypass grafting
B. For aortic valve replacement it is approximately 6 %
C. For mitral valve replacement it is approximately 4 %
D. For mitral valve repair it is 3%
E. For aortic valve replacement and coronary artery bypass grafting it is 6-8%

T F F T T

The mortality for aortic valve replacement is approximately 4 % and for mitral valve replacement approximately 6 %. These are based on both the North American and UK databases available for public access.

Q3 Which of the following are risk factors for increased rate of bioprosthetic valve calcification and resultant stenosis after implantation?

A. Older age at implantation

B. Chronic renal failure
C. Aortic valve position
D. Pregnancy
E. Thyrotoxicosis

F T F T F

There is some evidence of increased calcification at the mitral position, whilst other studies find no difference.

Q4   Which of the following statements regarding coronary artery fistulae are correct?

A. The majority arise from the left coronary artery
B. They are a complication of surgery for tetralogy of Fallot
C. They are associated with pulmonary atresia
D. They may be complicated by infective endocarditis
E. They must always be closed by either surgical ligation or embolisation

F T T T F

Most fistulae arise from the right coronary artery (60%) and terminate in the right side of the heart (90%). They may be associated with other congenital cardiac anomalies, most frequently critical pulmonary stenosis or atresia with an intact interventricular septum and with pulmonary artery branch stenosis, coarctation of the aorta, and aortic atresia. Although most often congenital, a coronary fistula rarely may arise as a consequence of surgical resection of obstructing right ventricular muscle bundles (as in tetralogy of Fallot), endomyocardial biopsy, or penetrating or blunt trauma.

Q5 Which of the following are features of carcinoid heart disease?

   A. Only carcinoid tumours that invade the liver usually result in pathological changes to the heart

   B. The cardiac manifestations are caused by the effects of 5-hydroxytryptamine (serotonin)

   C. It is characterised by the presence of densely calcific endocardial plaques

   D. Left sided valvar pathology occurs in a third of patients

   E. It has a 3 year survival of 30%

T T F F T

Ordinarily, the vasoactive tumour products are inactivated by the liver, lungs, and brain, but the presence of hepatic metastases may allow large quantities of these substances to reach the right side of the heart without being inactivated by the liver. The characteristic pathological findings are endocardial plaques of fibrous tissue that may involve the tricuspid valve, pulmonary valve, cardiac chambers, venae cavae, pulmonary artery, and coronary sinus. The fibrous tissue in the plaques results in distortion of the valves leading to either stenosis, regurgitation, or both. The preferential right heart involvement is most likely related to inactivation of the vasoactive substances by the lungs. In the 5–10% of cases with left sided valvar pathology, one should suspect bronchial carcinoid, or a patent foramen ovale.

Q6 Which of the following correctly describe papillary fibroelastoma?

   A. They are benign endocardial papillomas that predominantly affect the cardiac valves

   B. They are the second most common primary benign cardiac neoplasm

   C. They are a cause of sudden death

D. They are found mainly on the tricuspid or pulmonary valves, at the valvular free edges

E. Simple surgical excision with leaflet repair should not be attempted due to the likelihood of recurrence

T T T F F

Patients may present with chest pain, transient ischemic attacks or stroke, dyspnoea, or sudden death secondary to obstruction of the coronary ostia or embolisation. Embolic fragments may arise from the tumour itself or from platelet and fibrin clots that may form on its surface. They are found mainly on the aortic or mitral valves, away from the valvular free edges. Simple surgical excision with possible leaflet repair or valve replacement should be performed. Recurrence after complete surgical resection has not been reported.

Q7 Which of the following statements regarding the management of heart failure are true?

A. Cardiogenic shock is the most common cause of death for patients hospitalised with acute myocardial infarction

B. In patients in cardiogenic shock after acute myocardial infarction, survival at 30 days does not differ significantly between emergency revascularization (PCI or CABG) and initial medical stabilisation

C. The American College of Cardiology/American Heart Association guidelines for myocardial infarction recommend emergency revascularisation for patients younger than 75 years with cardiogenic shock

D. Autologous skeletal muscle-cell injections improve regional contractility in cell-transplanted infarcts and increase left ventricular ejection fraction, in patients with heart failure

E. Catheter based delivery of autologous bone marrow stem cells to affected myocardium has been associated with improved symptoms and function

T T T F T

The 'Should We Emergently Revascularize Occluded Coronaries for Cardiogenic Shock (SHOCK)' trial showed that emergency revascularisation by either coronary artery bypass grafting or angioplasty did not affect survival at 30 days but showed that there was a significant survival benefit with early revascularization at the 6- and 12-month follow-up. The 'Myoblast Autologous Grafting in Ischemic Cardiomyopathy (MAGIC)' trial used skeletal muscle cells and failed to reach its primary efficacy end point of improving local or global cardiac contractility in patients with ischaemic heart failure.

✓ Q8 Which of the following are correct regarding aortic stenosis?

A. It results in eccentric hypertrophy of the left ventricle
B. An audible fourth heart sound indicates the onset of left ventricular failure
C. Congenital bicuspid valves cause calcific aortic stenosis 4 times more frequently than acquired forms do
D. Associated angina is preferably treated with oral nitrates
E. Atrial fibrillation is preferably treated with digoxin

F F T F F

In aortic stenosis (AS) pressure overload in the left ventricle, over time, causes an increase in ventricular wall thickness (concentric hypertrophy). An audible fourth heart sound indicates the presence of left ventricular hypertrophy in severe stenosis. Nitroglycerin-induced syncope occurs more often in patients with AS than in those without AS. Atrial fibrillation in the setting of AS is considered an emergency and should be converted urgently in patients who are haemodynamically unstable.

Q9 Regarding deep sternal wound infections

A. They require a temperature of >38° C to make the diagnosis
B. They are more common in diabetic patients
C. They are more common in obese patients
D. The mortality from them remains as high as 10%-20%
E. The CRP is a poor guide in assessing the response to treatment

F T T T F

The CDC (Centre for Disease Control) definitions of nosocomial infections requires only at least one of - a temperature >38° C, purulent drainage, other evidence of infection of the deep tissue on direct examination. Independent risk factors after coronary artery bypass grafting were obesity, bilateral internal thoracic artery grafting, re-operation, and postoperative inotropic support.

Q10 Which of the following are true regarding mitral valve prolapse?

A. Patients with an isolated click have a general mortality rate that is increased by 15-20%
B. It is associated with Systemic lupus erythematosus.
C. ACE inhibitors halt the progression of mitral valve prolapse to mitral regurgitation
D. Mitral regurgitation is the most significant risk factor for sudden death, stroke, and endocarditis
E. Post stroke patients with mitral valve prolapse and regurgitation should receive aspirin

F T F T F

Significant mitral regurgitation in the setting of hypertension may be improved with the use of ACE inhibitors, but no evidence exists that it halts the progression to mitral regurgitation. Post stroke patients with mitral valve prolapse associated with atrial fibrillation, left atrial thrombus or regurgitation should receive long term anticoagulation with warfarin (class I evidence).

Q11 Which of the following are true regarding the Fontan procedure?

A. It consists of diversion of all of the systemic venous return to the pulmonary arteries, without using a subpulmonary ventricle
B. Protein-losing enteropathy occurs in up to half of post-operative Fontan patients
C. Pulmonary arterio-venous malformations are a cause of worsening cyanosis.
D. Development of dysrhythmias is unlikely to be related to an underlying haemodynamic cause
E. If permanent pacing is required, epicardial A-V sequential pacing should be used

T F T F T

Protein-losing enteropathy occurs in up to 10% of patients after the Fontan procedure. When dysrhythmias are present, an underlying haemodynamic cause should always be sought, and in particular, obstruction of the Fontan circuit needs to be excluded. If permanent pacing is required, epicardial A-V sequential pacing should be employed whenever possible to reduce the risk of thromboembolism.

Q12 Following tricuspid valve surgery

A. The patient may present with ST segment changes in leads II, III, and aVF postoperatively

B. The patient should be anticoagulated postoperatively for valve replacement

C. Epicardial pacing wires do not require to be placed at the end of the operation if the patient is in sinus rhythm

D. A patient manifesting tricuspid regurgitation due to carcinoid heart disease has a better outcome with repair than with replacement

E. Late survival is better with valve repair than with replacement

T F F F F

Most patients with tricuspid regurgitation are likely to receive a form of tricuspid valve repair. Valve replacement is more likely required in tricuspid stenosis and biological valves are used to avoid the need for anticoagulation.

Q13 Which of the following statements regarding doppler assessment of the cardiovascular system are true?

A. The Bernoulli equation (gradient $= 4V^2$) is used to calculate the pressure gradient across a valve

B. The peak tricuspid regurgitation velocity is used to calculate the mean pulmonary artery pressure

C. Measuring the area of the colour regurgitant jet is a semiquantitative method of estimating the severity of tricuspid regurgitation

D. The estimated cardiac output is based on the square of the measured radius of the aorta

E. Doppler estimates of the aortic peak gradient calculated using the simplified Bernoulli formula generally overestimate severity when compared with catheterisation peak-to-peak gradients

T F T T T

The distance from the baseline to the peak of the TR is measured (in centimeters) and expressed as velocity (V). It is then used to determine the gradient across the tricuspid valve (in millimeters of mercury) as $4V^2$. If V is 3 cm, therefore the calculated gradient is approximately 36 mm Hg. By adding the right atrial pressure (usually taken as 10 mm Hg) to this value, the systolic right ventricular and pulmonary arterial pressure can be determined in tricuspid regurgitation. Doppler estimates of cardiac output compare quite favourably with those obtained by other methods but any error in this measurement will be multiplied and may profoundly affect the resulting calculation.

Q14 Regarding the post-pericardiotomy syndrome

A. Symptoms usually develop within 1-6 weeks after surgery involving pericardiotomy
B. Anti-heart antibodies in high titre is a confirmatory diagnostic test
C. Patients manifest arthralgia
D. Low QRS amplitude on the ECG should alert to myocardial damage
E. Pre-cardiopulmonary bypass steroids reduce the risk of developing the condition

T T T F F

A temperature in a patient appearing well, malaise, chest pain, decreased appetite, dyspnoea and arthralgias may all consist of the syndrome. Tachycardia, a pericardial friction rub, a pleural friction rub and the accumulation of pericardial fluid and systemic fluid retention with hepatomegaly also occur. A 4-fold or greater rise in anti-heart antibodies is frequently associated. The ECG may show low QRS amplitude, especially with a large pericardial effusion. There is no evidence that pre-cardiopulmonary bypass steroids reduce the risk of developing the syndrome.

Q15 In infective endocarditis in children with congenital heart disease

    A. Staphylococcus aureus is the most frequent pathogen
    B. The most common associated abnormality is a PDA
    C. A VSD is a common site of infection
    D. Detection of vegetations by 2-dimensional echocardiography is absent in the majority of patients
    E. An aggressive surgical approach is not justified

F F T F F

Streptococcus viridans is the most frequent pathogen and staphylococcus aureus the second most frequent. Bicuspid aortic valve is the most common underlying heart disease occurring in approximately 30% of cases.

Q16 Regarding transposition of the great arteries

    A. It is the most common neonatal cyanotic congenital heart lesion
    B. It is associated with an intact ventricular septum 50% of the time
    C. In approximately 4% of patients, the coronary artery anatomy is abnormal
    D. It has a clear female predominance

E. An arterial switch procedure should be performed when the infant is younger than 4 weeks

T T F F T

In approximately one third of patients with TGA, the coronary artery anatomy is abnormal (left circumflex coronary arising from the right coronary artery in 22%, a single right coronary artery in 9.5%, a single left coronary artery in 3%, or inverted origin of the coronary arteries in 3%, representing the most common variants. It has a male predominance. The arterial switch procedure should be performed when the infant is younger than 4 weeks, as the left ventricle may not be able to handle systemic pressure postoperatively, if left too long connected to the low-pressure, low-resistance, pulmonary circulation.

Q17 Which of the following are correct regarding aortic regurgitation?

A. The incidence of sudden death in asymptomatic patients with normal left ventricular function is 0.2% per year
B. The incidence of sudden death in symptomatic patients or patients with impaired left ventricular function is between 6-10% per year
C. When acute causes dilation of the left ventricle
D. When chronic causes eccentric hypertrophy
E. The development of a third heart sound coincides with the onset of left ventricular dysfunction

T T F T T

Chronic aortic regurgitation causes eccentric hypertrophy, whilst pressure overload of the left ventricle, as occurs with aortic stenosis and systemic hypertension, causes concentric hypertrophy.

Q18 Cardiac myxomas

A. Are thought to arise from connective tissue cells in the subendocardium
B. Are more common in males
C. Are the most common primary cardiac tumour
D. Occur as a familial form (the Carney complex) in elderly females
E. Occurring sporadically recur after surgical resection in <5% of patients

T F T F T

Carney first described patients with myxomas, spotty pigmentation of skin and mucous membranes, and endocrine overactivity. This syndrome belongs to a group of genetic disorders, the lentiginoses, which include Peutz-Jeghers, LEOPARD, and Laugier-Hunziker syndromes. Cardiac myxomas occur in young females with this complex. The recurrence rate after surgery of familial patients is 20%.

Q19 Which of the following is true of pulmonary regurgitation?

A. When detected echocardiographically it is pathological
B. It is associated with a widely split S2
C. It is associated with the Graham Steell murmur when the PA systolic pressure is >60 mmHg
D. It occurs in connective tissue disorders
E. It is associated with reversed 'R' wave progression on the ECG

F T T T T

Increased right ventricular end-diastolic volume causes the right ventricular ejection time to be increased with P_2 delayed. This widens the normal split in S$_2$. The Graham Steell murmur is a high-pitched early diastolic murmur that is indicative of pulmonary hypertension.

Q20 Which of the following is true of truncus arteriosus?

A. Persistent left superior vena cava occurs in approximately 10%
B. The aortic arch is right sided in 25%
C. It has a 50% mortality in the first month
D. A ductus arteriosus is required to support the foetal circulation
E. Pulmonary blood flow typically is at least 3-fold higher than systemic blood flow

T T T F T

Because the common trunk originates from both the left and right ventricles, and pulmonary arteries arise directly from the common trunk, a ductus arteriosus is not required to support the foetal circulation. Outflow from both ventricles is directed into the common arterial trunk and hence pulmonary blood flow depends on the ratio between resistance to flow in the pulmonary and systemic vascular beds.

Q21 Atherosclerotic aortic aneurysms

A. Affect males more often than females
B. Are the commonest cause of an ascending aortic aneurysm
C. Are commonly associated with embolic phenomena
D. Are best demonstrated by aortography
E. May be treated by endovascular stenting

T F T F T

Atherosclerosis is the most common cause of thoracic aneurysms overall but not of the ascending aorta. The risk of aortography includes embolisation from atherosclerotic plaque and surface thrombus and thus carries a stroke risk. CT scans with contrast are a safer option. Endovascular stenting may be the only feasible option in patients who are considered unfit for surgery.

Q22 Which of the following statements regarding inflammatory and infective processes occurring on the heart valves are correct?

A. Libman-Sacks endocarditis is due to a fungus
B. When infective in origin, occur on the low pressure side of a valvular defect
C. Marantic endocarditis occurs in cachectic states
D. Xenogeneic aortic heart valve prostheses express high levels of integrins in contrast to native valves
E. LDL cholesterol levels influence the progression of aortic valve calcification

F T T F T

Libman-Sacks endocarditis is seen in SLE. Immunoglobulin superfamily adhesion molecules (ELAM-1, ICAM-1 and -2, CD34, CD44) but not integrins or selectins appear to be expressed in high levels, and thought to relate to immunological reactions that play a role in the degeneration of biological heart valve prostheses (J Heart Valve Dis. 2003; 12: 520-6.). The association between high LDL cholesterol levels and progression of aortic valve calcification has been studied using volumetric scoring on CT scans (Circulation. 2001; 104:1927.)

Q23 Which of the following are true regarding pulmonary hypertension?

A. It is defined by a mean pressure at rest exceeding 25 mm Hg
B. It is seen in transposition of the great arteries
C. Chronic obstructive airways disease is the most common cause of secondary pulmonary hypertension
D. It is associated with a loud P2
E. The median survival from the time of diagnosis is 2-3 years

T T T T F

Pulmonary hypertension is defined by a mean pressure at rest exceeding 25 mm Hg or at exercise exceeding 30 mmHg. It is seen in transposition of the great arteries due to increased pulmonary blood flow. Lung diseases that cause hypoxia cause pulmonary hypertension. Historically if untreated, the median survival from the time of diagnosis was 2-3 years, but the use of bosentan (an oral dual endothelin receptor antagonist) and other drugs shows a 3 year survival greater than 80%.

Q24 In a patient with mitral valve disease, valve repair

A. Has a higher mortality at the time of operation
B. Has a poorer late survival than replacement
C. Has a lower risk of thromboembolic phenomena than replacement
D. Is the preferred option in patients with a calcified mitral valve annulus
E. For mitral valve prolapse is only performed when mitral valve regurgitation is present

F F T F T

Mitral valve repair has a lower mortality at the time of operation (1- 2 %) as compared to 6-8% for replacement. Isolated mitral valve prolapse without regurgitation is common and occurs in approximately 1 in every 20 people. In the absence of regurgitation repair is not proven to impact upon survival.

Q25 Which of the following are true of congenital pulmonary stenosis?

A. Infundibular pulmonary stenosis occurs with Tetralogy of Fallot.
B. It is most often sub-valvar in type
C. In the Noonan syndrome it is associated with a bi-cuspid pulmonary valve
D. It is supravalvar when associated with maternal rubella infection
E. It may be associated with hypercalcaemia

T F T T T

Congenital pulmonary stenosis is valvar in 85%. Noonan syndrome is associated with heart disease in the majority, manifesting as pulmonary valve stenosis, pulmonary artery stenosis, septal defects and hypertrophic cardiomyopathy.

Q26 In a patient in septicaemic shock after a clam shell incision.

A. Extensive bleeding may occur due to depletion of fibrinogen levels
B. Extensive bleeding may occur due to depletion of platelet levels
C. Pulmonary oedema may occur
D. Hypotension should be treated with dobutamine
E. An empyema may be the underlying cause

T T T F T

In the context of the low systemic vascular resistance that is present in septicaemic shock the use of drugs such as dobutamine will result in further vasodilatation and compound the situation. If used to support cardiac function concomitant vasoconstrictors will likely need to be used in combination.

✓Q27 Regarding the aortic root and processes affecting it

A. The aortic root is normally 2 - 3.7 cm
B. The root is equivalent in diameter to the sino-tubulo junction
C. Once an aortic root abscess is detected surgery is deferred till antibiotics control the infection and negative blood cultures are obtained
D. The development of heart block on the surface ECG a week after aortic valve replacement is highly suggestive of a root abscess
E. Sinus of Valsalva dilatation is independently related to male gender

T F F T T

The aortic root is 10-15% greater in diameter than the sino-tubular junction, which can increase in diameter with increasing age and in disease. Once an aortic root abscess is detected, urgent surgery is required as antibiotics alone will fail to control the infection. Debridement of all infected and devitalised tissue is the mainstay of the surgical treatment. Delayed lengthening of the PR interval or development of heart block on the surface ECG in the pre-echocardiographic era were considered as highly suggestive of a root abscess after surgery.

Q28 Which of the following are correct regarding ventricular assist devices?

A. Continuous flow pumps are referred to as second generation ventricular assist devices
B. Third generation ventricular assist devices suspend the impeller in the pump using bearings
C. Early institution of circulatory support is associated with improved outcomes
D. A percutaneous left ventricular assist device is indicated in patients with a postinfarction ventricular septal defect as a bridge to surgery.
E. A survival advantage in patients receiving a ventricular assist device for long term management of heart failure is not clearly established

T F T F F

First generation ventricular assist devices were "pulsatile" and blood was alternately sucked into the pump and ejected out. Third generation ventricular assist devices suspend the impeller using either hydrodynamic or electromagnetic suspension. A VSD is deemed to be a relative contraindication for a percutaneous left ventricular assist device because of the risk of right-to-left shunting with subsequent hypoxaemia. The landmark 'Randomized Evaluation of Mechanical Assistance for The Treatment of Congestive Heart Failure (REMATCH)' trial, specifically compared the survival of patients receiving the Heartmate VAD with those treated with optimal medical therapy and showed survival at one year to be 52% in the device group and 25% in the medical therapy group, with the rates at two years being 23% and 8%, respectively.

Q29 Which of the following are true regarding the tricuspid valve?

    A. It has a well formed annulus

    B. The antero-septal commisure is supported by the medial papillary muscle

    C. A De-vega procedure consists of an anterior plicating suture

    D. Atrio-ventricular conduction may be damaged by a De-vega procedure

    E. Tricuspid regurgitation may be treated by bicuspidisation of the tricuspid valve by suturing the septal to the anterior leaflet

F T T F F

The annulus is not uniformly thick throughout its circumference and it is contributed to by several elements- the right fibrous trigone where it faces the tricuspid valve, right and left long, tapering subendocardial fibrous bands - the fila coronaria - passing laterally from the right fibrous trigone and a very thin layer of connective tissue between the distal ends of the fila coronaria laterally.

Q30 Which of the following statements regarding DiGeorge syndrome are false?

    A. It is associated with hypercalcaemia

    B. It is associated with abnormalities in the migration of neural crest cells to the region of the pharyngeal pouches

    C. It is present in approximately 30-35% of patients with truncus arteriosus

    D. It is the most frequent contiguous gene deletion syndrome in humans

    E. Children with the condition having cardiac surgery should have non-irradiated blood products

F T T T F

It is associated with hypocalcaemia due to hypoparathyroidism. The DiGeorge anomaly has traditionally been described as abnormal development of the third and fourth pharyngeal pouches but defects involving the first to sixth pouches are also known to occur, thought to be related to defective migration of neural crest cells to the region of the pharyngeal pouches. Fluorescent in situ hybridization (FISH) probes show that over 90% patients with the DiGeorge anomaly have a microdeletion of 22q11.21 through 22q11.23, spanning approximately 2 megabases in length. The utmost care must be taken to avoid non-irradiated blood products due to the associated immune deficiency.

Q31　Which of the following statements about prosthetic valve endocarditis are correct?

A. Early prosthetic aortic valve endocarditis occurs within 60 days of implantation
B. Early prosthetic valve endocarditis is usually caused by staphylococcus and enterococcus
C. Late prosthetic valve endocarditis in bioprosthetic valves usually involves the sewing ring
D. It should be treated with vancomycin and gentamycin, empirically pending blood cultures
E. Overall mortality for late prosthetic valve endocarditis is <5 %

T T F T F

Late prosthetic valve endocarditis in bioprosthetic valves usually involves the leaflets whilst in mechanical valves it involves the sewing ring. Although overall mortality for late prosthetic valve endocarditis is 20 % (contributed to by the HACEK group and staphylococci), it is most often caused by streptococci, which have a mortality rate < 5%.

✓Q32 Which of the following are true of ischaemic mitral insufficiency?

A. It is irreversible without valvular intervention
B. The antero-posterior diameter of the mitral annulus exceeds the transverse diameter in systole
C. When secondary to papillary muscle rupture it occurs two to seven days after the infarct
D. When due to a ruptured papillary muscle it involves the anterior papillary muscle more commonly than the posterior muscle.
E. Right heart catheterisation shows prominent "v" waves

F T T F T

Ischaemic mitral insufficiency may be seen with acute ischaemia, a setting in which the regurgitation typically resolves after the ischaemia resolves. In ischaemic mitral insufficiency, the annulus is dilated in its muscular posterior portion resulting in an antero-posterior diameter that exceeds the transverse diameter in systole. The posterior papillary muscle is involved more commonly than is the anterior muscle.

Q33 Which of the following are true of Cor Triatriatum?

A. It is a condition where a right atrium, left atrium and a doubly committed common atrium co-exist
B. It is associated with a persistent left superior vena cava
C. In cor triatriatum sinistrum the ECG shows right axis deviation

D. The location of the atrial appendage differentiates cor triatriatum from a supra-valvular mitral stenosis
E. In the majority surgical intervention is not required

F T T T F

It is a congenital anomaly in which either the left atrium (cor triatriatum sinistrum) or right atrium (cor triatriatum dextrum) is divided into two parts by a tissue fold, or fibromuscular band. Usually, the proximal/upper portion of the atrium receives venous blood, and the distal portion connects with the atrio-ventricular valve. In cor triatriatum sinistrum the ECG may show right axis deviation due to right ventricular hypertrophy and needs to be differentiated from supra-valvular mitral stenosis. In cor triatriatum, the left atrial appendage is in the same chamber with the mitral valve ring, distal to the atrial membrane. Most require surgery at a young age, usually before the age of one year.

Q34 Which of the following are correct regarding postinfarction ventricular septal defects?

A. Approximately 40% occur with infarction of the anterior wall
B. The surgical mortality rate for anterior defects is greater than for posterior defects
C. An IABP offers the most important means of temporary haemodynamic support
D. Ventricular aneurysms are commonly associated with them
E. Right heart catheterisation helps differentiate them from acute ischaemic mitral regurgitation

F F T T T

Approximately 60% occur with infarction of the anterior wall. The surgical mortality rate for anterior defects is 10-15% and for posterior defects is 30-35%. Some series show an association with ventricular aneurysms in approximately half of the patients. Right heart catheterisation helps differentiate them from acute ischaemic mitral regurgitation, by the absence of a 'v' wave and by the presence of an oxygen concentration step up between the right atrium and the pulmonary artery.

Q35 Which of the following are true regarding atrial fibrillation?

A. With a normal sized atrium is due to macro-re-entry circuits
B. It is the commonest dysrhythmia following pneumonectomy
C. The annual risk for stroke in patients with chronic atrial fibrillation is 5%
D. The AFFIRM study showed rhythm conrol to be superior to rate control in preventing strokes
E. Cardioversion should not be performed without adequate anticoagulation in patients who have been in atrial fibrillation for more than 48 hours

F T T F T

When the atrium is 'normal' (normal size and not appearing diseased), the pathophysiology of atrial fibrillation is usually of focal triggers of enhanced automaticity. The AFFIRM study showed no difference in stroke risk in patients who converted to sinus rhythm with anti-arrhythmic treatment, when compared to those who had only rate control.

Q36 Which are correct satatements regarding stentless valves?

A. For a given external diameter, the internal diameter of a stentless valve is 2 to 4 mm larger than a stent mounted valve

B. They may only be used in the subcoronary position
C. They should only be used if the difference in diameters of the annulus and sino-tubular junction is greater than 10%
D. The muscular portion of the stentless xenograft valve should be aligned with the non-coronary cusp
E. The proximal suture line is placed in the annular position

T F F T F

Implantation requirements can vary between individual stentless valve types ranging from subcoronary implant to a choice of either a subcoronary, cylindrical or a root replacement implant. Stentless valves should only be used if the difference in diameters of the annulus and sino-tubular junction is less than 10%. The lower suture line is placed in the sub-annular position as a single horizontal plane.

Q37 Which of the following are true of a double aortic arch?

A. It is the most common type of vascular ring
B. The most common form of double aortic arch is a left (anterior) dominant arch
C. It produces a reverse 'S' sign on antero-posterior contrast oesophagography
D. The surgical approach to a double aortic arch is through a left thoracotomy
E. Persistence of a child's noisy breathing on extubation after surgical division indicates incomplete division of the ring

T F T T F

The most common form of double aortic arch is a right (posterior) dominant arch. The reverse 'S' sign is produced by the relative indentations caused by the right arch which is higher and the left arch which is lower. It may take months for the child's noisy breathing to completely disappear as the tracheo-bronchomalacia caused by the rings needs to resolve.

Q38 Regarding hypertrophic obstructive cardiomyopathy

A. It is associated with symmetrical septal hypertrophy
B. It is associated with a ratio of septal wall thickness to the posterior wall > 1.5
C. Myocardial bridging of the LAD is common
D. DDD pacing produces a significant increase in cardiac output
E. It may require mitral valve surgery

F T T T T

It is associated with asymmetrical septal hypertrophy. In addition to obstructing blood flow, the thickened wall may distort a leaflet of the mitral valve, causing mitral regurgitation. In over half the cases the disease is hereditary.

Q39 Patient-prosthesis mismatch

A. Is best defined by the geometric orifice area of the valve
B. Is severe when the indexed effective orifice area is less than $0.65 \text{ cm}^2/\text{m}^2$
C. Is also influenced by the patient's functional state
D. May manifest as shortness of breath
E. Is more likely to occur with a mechanical valve prosthesis than with a stented bioprosthesis of the same external diameter

F T F T F

The geometric orifice area is a measurement derived from the internal diameter of the prosthesis and measured in vitro by the valve manufacturer. It has been shown to overestimate the 'functional area' of a valve prosthesis. Following the introduction of echocardiography, a more reliable parameter has been validated in clinical practice and is termed the effective orifice area. The concept of patient-prosthesis mismatch is considered to occur when the indexed effective orifice area is less than 0.85 cm^2/m^2 to 0.75 cm^2/m^2. Mechanical valve prostheses have a more favourable relationship between their external diameter and the effective orifice area when compared to a stented bioprosthesis.

Q40 Which statements are true of secundum atrial septal defects?

A. 80% of all atrial septal defects are ostium secundum defects
B. Deficiency of the septum primum is the commonest cause of a ostium secundum atrial septal defect
C. Pulmonary hypertension develops by adolescence
D. Fixed splitting of S_2 is present
E. The defect is better visualised with the use of transthoracic echocardiography than with transoesophageal echocardiography

T T F T F

Pulmonary hypertension is unusual before 20 years of age, and is seen in half of individuals with an atrial septal defect above the age of 40 years. Fixed splitting of the second heart sound occurs because the extra blood return during inspiration gets equalised between the left and right atrium due to the communication that exists between the atria in the presence of an atrial septal defect.

Q41 Regarding aortic stenosis and coronary artery disease

    A. Angina in patients with aortic stenosis is nearly always associated with significant coronary disease

    B. In adults with severe aortic stenosis, 25% have significant coronary artery disease

    C. Most patients with coronary artery disease do not have aortic stenosis

    D. A peak transvalvar aortic gradient of 30 mmHg is an indication for aortic valve replacement in a patient having coronary artery bypass grafting

    E. A peak transvalvar aortic gradient of 20 mmHg in a patient with impaired left ventricular function is a contraindication for aortic valve replacement in a patient having coronary artery bypass grafting

T F T T F

In adults with severe aortic stenosis, 50% have significant coronary artery disease. ACC/AHA 2006 Guidelines for the Management of Patients with Valvular Heart Disease recommends that patients with intermediate aortic valve gradients (30 to 50 mm Hg mean gradient at catheterisation or transvalvular velocity of 3 to 4 m per second by Doppler echocardiography) who are undergoing CABG may warrant AVR at the time of revascularisation. As the pressure gradient across a stenotic valve is related to the valve orifice area and the transvalvular flow in the presence of depressed cardiac output, low pressure gradients may be obtained in patients with significant aortic stenosis. Dobutamine stress echocardiography is reasonable to evaluate patients with low-flow/low-gradient AS and LV dysfunction. If there is latent ventricular reserve the gradient will then increase.

Q42 Regarding partial anomalous pulmonary venous connection

    A. The anomalous veins drain into the chest wall venous system
    B. Anomalous drainage from the left lung is twice as common as from the right lung
    C. The commonest type is that associated with a sinus venosus type atrial septal defect
    D. It is associated with the scimitar syndrome
    E. Oxygen sampling may identify the location of an anomalous vein

F F T T T

The anomalous veins drain into the systemic venous return, and anomalous drainage from the right lung is twice as common as from the left lung. The most common form is one in which a right upper pulmonary vein connects to the right atrium or the superior vena cava and is almost always associated with a sinus venosus type of atrial septal defect. The Scimitar syndrome (pulmonary venolobar syndrome) consists of abnormal right pulmonary venous drainage to the inferior vena cava and an abnormal arterial supply of the right lung from the descending aorta and with right lung malformation/hypoplasia.

Q43 Which of the following are true regarding mitral annular calcification?

    A. It occurs in about 6% of persons >60 years of age
    B. It occurs predominantly in men
    C. Chronic mitral regurgitation may occur due to mitral annular calcification
    D. Mitral annular calcification is associated with coronary artery disease
    E. It is associated with sick sinus syndrome

T F T T F

Mitral annular calcification occurs predominantly in women. Mitral regurgitation due to mitral annular calcification prevents annular contraction in systole, and may limit valve leaflet closure but is rarely of haemodynamic significance. Calcification may involve the conduction system, causing degrees of atrioventricular block.

Q44 Which are true regarding pulmonary vascular disease?

A. Primary pulmonary hypertension is more common than secondary pulmonary hypertension
B. Primary pulmonary hypertension is characterised by an elevated pulmonary wedge pressure
C. Pulmonary hypertension secondary to fibrotic lung disease is severe and relentless
D. Hypoxic pulmonary vasoconstriction contributes to its occurrence in chronic obstructive lung disease
E. Pulmonary thromboembolism is the most common cause of pulmonary vascular disease

F F F T T

Primary pulmonary hypertension is characterised by an elevated pulmonary artery pressure and normal pulmonary wedge pressure. In pulmonary hypertension secondary to fibrotic lung disease patients do not tend to develop pulmonary hypertension until very late as only a part of the pulmonary arterial tree is involved until the disease is advanced.

Q45 Which of the following cardiac tumours occur primarily in the paediatric age group?

A. Rhabdomyoma
B. Fibroma
C. Purkinje tumours
D. Sarcoma
E. Hamartoma

T T T F T

Rhabdomyomas, accounting for about 20% of cardiac tumours, occur in children or infants and are associated with tuberous sclerosis, adenoma sebaceum of the skin, kidney tumours and dysrhythmias. Fibromas, which also develop in the myocardium or the endocardium, mostly occur on the valves of the heart. Teratomas of the pericardium, not uncommonly attached to the base of the great vessels, usually occur in infants. Malignant cardiac tumours occur mostly in children and include angiosarcomas, which account for about a third of all malignant cardiac tumours. They start usually on the right side of the heart. In addition fibrosarcomas, rhabdomyosarcomas and liposarcomas occur.

Q46 Which of the following are true of bacterial endocarditis?

A. Large numbers of white blood cells are seen when vegetations are viewed under a microscope
B. It occurs commonly in patients with secundum atrial septal defects
C. It is caused by a deficiency in complement activity
D. The most common location for endocarditis in patients with ventricular septal defects is on the septal leaflet of the tricuspid valve
E. Janeway lesions are tender macules

F F F T F

The reason for the absence of white blood cells in vegetations is not entirely clear, but thought to be due to the bacteria being deep within the vegetations, which can be dense in nature, thus restricting the migration of white cells. The shunt across a secundum atrial septal defect is a low pressure one and hence carries a low risk of infective endocarditis. Micro-organisms that most commonly produce endocarditis (S aureus, S viridans, and enterococci) resist the bactericidal action of complement. Janeway lesions are painless macules, in contrast to Osler nodes that are tender nodules.

Q47 Which of the following are true of coarctation of the aorta?

A. The male-to-female ratio is 1:2
B. It is the commonest cardiac defect associated with Turner syndrome
C. It is associated with Berry aneurysms of the circle of Willis
D. A resting gradient across the coarctation > 20 mm Hg is an indication for repair
E. It may require an infusion of prostaglandin E1 at birth

F T T T T

The male-to-female ratio is 2:1. When presenting at birth prostaglandin E1 (0.05-0.15 mcg/kg/min) is infused intravenously to open the ductus arteriosus.

Q48 Regarding ventricular re-modelling procedures

A. The Bastista procedure attempts to specifically restore ventricular contour
B. The Bastista procedure is associated with good clinical improvement in patients' morbidity and mortality
C. The Dor procedure attempts specifically to restore ventricular contour
D. The Dor procedure attempts to restore the left ventricular cavity to a circular shape
E. They are performed concomitantly with coronary artery bypass grafting

F F T F T

The Bastista procedure does not attempt specifically to restore ventricular contour, and despite improvement in physiology did not show clear clinical benefits. The Dor procedure involves placing an endoventricular circular purse string suture at the base of the infarcted ventricle. It helps restore a more normal oval curvature of the ventricle. The remaining ventricular defect is closed with a pericardial patch.

Q49 Select the correct statements regarding Marfan Syndrome

A. It is an autosomal recessive disorder
B. Reduced levels of fibrillin-1 occur impairing the formation of elastic fibers
C. Decreased transforming growth factor beta (TGFβ) activity occurs
D. It is associated with pectus excavatum
E. It is a risk factor for spontaneous pneumothorax

F T F T T

Is an autosomal dominant disorder that has been linked to a defect in the Fibrillin-1 gene on chromosome 15. Fibrillin-1 binds TGFβ, inactivating it. In Marfan syndrome, reduced levels of fibrillin-1 allow TGFβ over activity.

Q50 Which of the following correctly describes annuloaortic ectasia?

A. It occurs in association with Takayasu arteritis
B. It is associated with polycystic kidney disease
C. It causes aortic regurgitation
D. When due to Marfan syndrome is differentiated from others having the condition by the presence of cystic medial necrosis
E. It is associated wit an increased diameter of the aortic root in relatives of almost half of the patients

T T T F T

Cystic medial degeneration manifests in annuloaortic ectasia, whether due to Marfan syndrome or not. An increased diameter of the aortic root is found in relatives of almost half of the patients who have the condition. However, there is no difference in elastin and collagen concentration between the familial and non-familial cases.

Q51 Which are correct statements regarding aortic valve repair?

A. When performed for aortic regurgitation a repair is complemented by aortic annuloplasty
B. A functional aortic annuloplasty consists of placing a annuloplasty ring in the subcoronary position
C. It is not suitable for rheumatic aortic valve incompetence due to cusp retraction

D. Regurgitation due to Arantius nodule hypertrophy can be treated with surgically shaving off the nodules
E. It is not suitable for adult patients with aortic regurgitation resulting from a congenitally bicuspid aortic valve

T F F T F

An aortic annuloplasty consists of subcommisural plicating sutures. The aortic valve may be repaired in incompetence due to cusp retraction of rheumatic origin with cusp extension using pericardium. A congenitally bicuspid aortic valve with prolapse of one of the cusps (more often the anterior) is particularly amenable to repair if the other cusp is not diseased.

Q52 Regarding cerebral protection in aortic surgery

A. Cerebral metabolism is reduced approximately 5% to 7% for each degree centigrade
B. Deep hypothermic circulatory arrest at 15° C eliminates the metabolic demands of the brain
C. Moderate levels of hypothermia, in contrast to deep hypothermia, permit a shorter total perfusion time
D. Retrograde cerebral perfusion is used at flow rates that maintain central venous pressure in the range of 15 to 25 mm Hg
E. Antegrade selective cerebral perfusion during moderate hypothermia (25°C) requires a perfusion volume of 10 ml/Kg/min

T F T T T

Cerebral metabolism in humans decreases exponentially with decreasing temperature. Despite the reduction in cerebral metabolism and oxygen requirement with profound hypothermia, there is still an ongoing, continuous need of substrates in the brain.

The human cerebral metabolic rate is still 17% of baseline at 15°C and the safe duration of circulatory arrest only 29 minutes (McCullough et al. Ann Thorac Surg 1999; 67: 1895-1899). Tanaka and colleagues suggest that the safe range of flow rates for cerebral perfusion during moderate hypothermia (25°C) is at least 50% of the physiologic level with a perfusion pressure ≥ 30 mm Hg.

Q53 Regarding Double Outlet Right Ventricle (DORV)

A. The aorta and main pulmonary artery are levo-rotated from the normal arrangement
B. The commonest type of ventricular septal defect seen in DORV is subaortic
C. A sub-pulmonary ventricular septal defect without pulmonary stenosis results in a cyanotic child
D. A subpulmonary ventricular septal defect with pulmonary outflow tract obstruction is managed with the arterial switch operation
E. Severe cyanosis during early infancy in the presence of pulmonary stenosis is best managed with a Blalock-Taussig shunt

F T T F T

The aorta and main pulmonary artery are dextro-rotated, often to lie side by side. In the DORV with a sub-pulmonary VSD without pulmonary stenosis, called the Taussig-Bing anomaly, oxygenated blood from the left ventricle is directed into the pulmonary artery, while de-oxygenated blood that returns to the right ventricle is directed into the aorta to give a physiology similar to patients with complete transposition of the great arteries. A sub-pulmonary VSD with pulmonary outflow tract obstruction is managed with a Rastelli repair, creating an intra-ventricular tunnel to baffle left ventricular blood to the aorta and placing a right ventricular-pulmonary artery conduit.

Q54 Which of the following are true regarding the Ross Procedure?

A. It is the replacement of the patient's diseased aortic valve with his/her own pulmonary valve
B. Longevity of the pulmonary autograft in the aortic position is superior to that of a porcine bioprosthesis
C. The pulmonary valve has the potential to grow as the child grows
D. It requires long term anticoagulation
E. It is useful in young patients with Marfan's syndrome

T T T F F

Anticoagulation is not required as with mechanical valves and thus patients can lead an active life without the risks associated with anticoagulant therapy. The Ross procedure is not indicated for patients with Marfan's syndrome, or other diseases that cause aortic root enlargement, as the underlying connective tissue disorder also affects the transferred pulmonary autograft.

Q55 Which of the following are true regarding carotid artery disease?

A. Early carotid artery wall disease is a predictor for coronary atherosclerosis
B. Intravenous digital angiography provides good resolution of the carotid bifurcation
C. Asymptomatic carotid stenosis carries a stroke risk of approximately 2% per year

D. The ACAS trial addressed asymptomatic stenosis in patients over 79 years of age
E. The benefit of carotid endarterectomy in symptomatic patients is demonstrated in prospective randomised trials

T F T F T

Intravenous digital angiography does not provide sufficient resolution of the carotid bifurcation. Imaging of the carotid bifurcation is performed using colour duplex scanning which is accurate and sensitive, providing information on the degree of stenosis and plaque morphology. The ACAS trial addressed asymptomatic stenoses in patients under 79 years of age. The benefit of carotid endarterectomy in symptomatic patients was demonstrated in both the NASCET (North American Symptomatic Carotid Endarterectomy Trial) and ECST (European Carotid Surgery Trial), both prospectively randomised trials.

√ Q56 Regarding aneurysms of the descending thoracic aorta

A. They are mostly atherosclerotic in aetiology
B. Patients who are awaiting the second stage after an elephant trunk repair are vulnerable to postoperative paraplegia
C. The aorta is cross-clamped just beyond the left subclavian artery for Crawford types III and IV aneurysms
D. Repair with a Gott shunt requires systemic heparinisation
E. Endoluminal graft placement has a greater incidence of neurological complications than does open surgery

T T F F F

Patients who have had an elephant trunk repair must be observed for signs of paraplegia because the telescoped sleeve in the descending aorta may obstruct the ostia of spinal arteries. The aorta is cross-clamped either just beyond the left subclavian or between the left carotid and left subclavian for Crawford types I and II but more distally for Crawford types III and IV. An external Gott shunt does not require systemic heparinisation as its heparin-coated wall prevents clotting. Endoluminal graft placement has an equal, if not less, incidence of neurological complications.

⌐ Q57 Which are true statements regarding traumatic aortic injury?

A. Ninety percent of thoracic aortic injuries occur in the region of the aortic isthmus
B. Traumatic false aneurysms result when the adventitia and media are disrupted but the intima remains intact and bulges outward through the defect
C. Chest radiography is the first screening test for aortic injury
D. The presence of a mediastinal haematoma indicates the presence of a traumatic aortic injury
E. Approximately 20 % of patients with untreated traumatic injury of the aorta survive long enough to form a chronic pseudoaneurysm

T F T F F

The isthmus is the portion of the proximal descending thoracic aorta between the origin of the left subclavian artery and the site of attachment of the ligamentum arteriosum. Traumatic false aneurysms result when the intima and media are disrupted and the adventitia bulges outward yet remains intact. Mediastinal haematoma may result from causes other than aortic injury, such as fractures of the lower cervical or upper thoracic vertebrae. Only 2% of patients with untreated traumatic injury of the aorta survive long enough to form a chronic pseudoaneurysm.

Q58 Which of the following are true of cardiac allograft rejection?

    A. Depletion of CD4[+] T cells in cardiac allograft recipients prolongs allograft survival

    B. CMV infection in cardiac transplant recipients is associated with an increased incidence of rejection

    C. Cardiac allograft vasculopathy is the major cause of morbidity and mortality in the first year after transplantation

    D. Acute cardiac allograft rejection is diagnosed by right ventricular endomyocardial biopsy

    E. Cardiac allograft vasculopathy is diagnosed by cardiac catheterisation with intravascular ultrasound

T T F T T

CMV infection in cardiac transplant recipients is associated with more frequent rejection, graft atherosclerosis, and death. In the first year acute cellular rejection and infection remain the most common causes of morbidity and mortality. Thereafter cardiac allograft vasculopathy as a result of chronic vascular rejection is the major cause of morbidity and mortality.

Q59 Ebstein's Anomaly

    A. Causes cyanosis

    B. Is associated with an atrial septal defect

    C. Presents as a supraventricular tachycardia

    D. Does not require antibiotic prophylaxis for endocarditis

    E. In a new born with a severely regurgitant valve requires early corrective surgery

T T T F F

If the tricuspid valve is severely displaced and regurgitant, congestion of the right atrium occurs, and elevates right atrial pressure. In the presence of an ASD, a right atrium to left atrium shunt will occur manifesting as cyanosis. An atrial septal defect is present almost 90% of the time. Supraventricular tachycardia may occur whether or not they have Wolff-Parkinson-White syndrome (present in 10 to 25%). Children with Ebstein's anomaly are at increased risk for subacute bacterial endocarditis. A Blalock-Taussig shunt in the neonatal period to improve pulmonary blood flow, and corrective surgery to repair or replace the tricuspid valve and close the atrial septal defect when the child is older, is the likely approach.

Q60 Which of the following are true regarding aortic dissection?

A. Men are twice as likely to be affected than women
B. A Stanford Type A aortic dissection spares the ascending aorta
C. Both DeBakey type I and DeBakey type II dissections involve the ascending aorta
D. Aortic dissections occur in otherwise healthy women during the first trimester of pregnancy
E. With successful surgery the 10 year survival is approximately 40% to 50%

T F T F T

A Stanford Type A aortic dissection involves the ascending aorta whilst a Type B spares it. A DeBakey type I dissection involves all sections of the thoracic and abdominal aorta, whilst a DeBakey type II involves only the ascending thoracic aorta. A DeBakey type III spares the ascending aorta. Aortic dissections occur in otherwise healthy women during the third trimester of pregnancy not the first.

Q61 Which of the following are correct regarding interrupted aortic arch?

    A. The most common site of interruption is distal to the left subclavian artery

    B. It is associated with a large ventricular septal defect in 70-90% of neonates

    C. It is associated with DiGeorge syndrome

    D. Sudden decompensation is likely if closure of the ductus arteriosus occurs

    E. May require re-operation in later life for subaortic stenosis

F T T T T

The most common site of interruption is between the left common carotid and left subclavian arteries. An interrupted aortic arch often occurs in association with other heart problems such as a ventricular septal defect, truncus arteriosus, transposition of the great arteries and aortic stenosis. In order to prevent sudden deterioration and maintain blood supply to the lower body, it is important to keep the ductus arteriosus open until surgery using an infusion of prostaglandin E2. In some patients, subaortic stenosis can occur needing re-operation. Also coarctation may develop at the aortic anastomotic site over time requiring balloon angioplasty or even re-operation.

Q62 Which of the following are true of a patent ductus arteriosus?

    A. It is associated with large birth weight

    B. A continuous murmur is typically heard, loudest at the left upper chest

    C. It is associated with congenital rubella

    D. Prophylaxis against infective endocarditis is not required

    E. It leads to pulmonary hypertension peaking in the fourth decade

F T T F F

Patent ductus arteriosus is associated with prematurity. A continuous murmur described as machinery in nature occurs due to a left to right shunt across the patent ductus and may be accentuated in systole. Prophylaxis against infective endocarditis is recommended as it connects a high pressure to a low pressure system, a situation that increases the risk of endocarditis. An increased incidence of elevated pulmonary vascular resistance and pulmonary hypertension occurs if closed in those older than 3 years and manifests much earlier than the fourth decade in all but the most restrictive connections between the systemic and pulmonary arterial systems.

Q63 Which of the following are true regarding the electrocardiogram?

A. The normal axis is -30° to +90°
B. The earliest electrocardiographic finding resulting from acute myocardial infarction is ST segment elevation
C. The normal PR interval is usually 0.12 to 0.20 seconds
D. The QT interval is measured from the beginning of the QRS complex to the beginning of the T wave
E. Prominent U waves are seen in hypokalaemia

T F T F T

The earliest electrocardiographic finding resulting from acute myocardial infarction is the hyperacute T wave. The PR interval is measured from the beginning of the P wave to the beginning of the QRS complex and is usually 0.12 to 0.20 seconds. The QT interval is measured from the beginning of the QRS complex to the end of the T wave and is usually about 0.40 seconds.

Q64 Which of the following are true regarding Tetralogy of Fallot?

A. It is a result of anterior malalignment of the conal septum
B. It is associated with a right-sided aortic arch, in 25% of patients
C. It is associated with a bicuspid pulmonary valve in 30-40% of patients
D. The mainstay in the treatment of hypercyanotic episodes is oxygen
E. A Blalock-Taussig shunt is performed as the first step in surgical management

T T T F F

Anterior malalignment of the conal septum results in a VSD, pulmonary stenosis, and an overriding aorta. Hypercyanotic episodes are thought to occur secondary to infundibular spasm/decreased SVR causing increased right-to-left shunting at the VSD leading to diminished pulmonary blood flow, and a limited response to oxygen. A Blalock-Taussig shunt is not normally performed unless complicating factors, such as the presence of severe pulmonary atresia, make it disirable to defer definitive sugery for when the child is older.

Q65 Regarding the surgical management of ascending aortic aneurysms

A. They may be treated with an interposition aortic graft
B. The re-implantation method of valve sparing root replacement involves re-implanting the scalloped native valve into the Dacron graft
C. The re-modeling method of valve sparing root replacement involves scalloping the Dacron graft
D. Marfan syndrome patients are best treated with tube graft replacement alone

E. The risk of air embolism is reduced by flooding the surgical field with carbon dioxide

T T T F T

Ascending aortic aneurysms with a normal aortic valve, annulus, and sinuses of Valsalva are managed with a tube graft from the sino-tubular junction to the origin of the innominate artery. The re-modelling method involves resecting the aneurysmal sinus tissue while maintaining the tissue along the valve leaflets and scalloping the Dacron graft to form new sinuses to remodel the root. The extent of the structural pathology of Marfan syndrome involves the aortic valve, annulus, and aorta, and these patients should have minimal residual tissue left behind to reduce the risk of recurrent aneurysm formation. Thus they should have an aortic root replacement when otherwise suitable.

Q66 Which of the following correctly describes atrio-ventricular septal defects?

A. They are associated with fixed splitting of the second heart sound
B. Usually they are associated with a cleft in the anterior mitral valve leaflet
C. A complete atrio-ventricular defect is more common than a partial atrio-ventricular defect in patients without Down syndrome
D. With a partial atrioventricular septal defect the anterior and posterior bridging leaflets are fused
E. The AV node is displaced anteriorly

T T F F F

Typically, the cleft in the mitral valve directs blood through the atrial defect into the right atrium causing its enlargement. Partial atrio-ventricular defect, as opposed to complete atrio-ventricular defect, of the ostium primum type is more common in patients without Down syndrome. The AV node is usually displaced posteriorly (originating in the posterior wall of the RA) as is the bundle of His which skirts the lower margin of the VSD. With a partial atrio-ventricular septal defect the mitral and tricuspid annuli are separate and hence no bridging leaflet is present. With both an intermediate atrio-ventricular septal defect and a complete atrio-ventricular septal defect there is a single valve annulus. The anterior and posterior bridging leaflets are fused in an intermediate defect whilst in a complete defect the anterior and posterior bridging leaflets are not fused but have contributions from both the tricuspid and mitral valves.

Q67 Cardiac re-synchronisation therapy

A. Is indicated for patients with symptomatic heart failure resulting from diastolic dysfunction
B. Is contraindicated in the presence of bundle branch block
C. Improves exercise capacity
D. In conjunction with an implantable defibrillator reduces mortality more than cardiac re-synchronisation therapy alone
E. Causes a significant reduction in cardiac cause mortality

F F T T F

Cardiac re-synchronisation therapy is indicated for patients with symptomatic heart failure resulting from systolic dysfunction. In approximately 30% of patients with heart failure, an abnormality in the heart's electrical conducting system (called an "intraventricular conduction delay" or bundle branch block) causes the two ventricles to beat in an asynchronous fashion. It is these patients who are likely to benefit from re-synchronisation. The COMPANION trial showed that patients receiving either kind of CRT device had more than a 20% reduction in the composite endpoint of the study (i.e., total hospitalisations and death from any cause). Patients who received cardiac re-synchronisation therapy plus a defibrillator showed a 36% reduction in mortality, whilst those who received cardiac re-synchronisation therapy without the defibrillator showed a trend toward a 24% reduction in mortality, though this was not statistically significant. There is no conclusive evidence on reduction in cardiac cause mortality.

Q68 Which of the following are true in aortic stenosis?

A. In severe aortic stenosis, the left atrial pressure waveform demonstrates a large 'a' wave
B. The subendocardium is susceptible to myocardial ischaemia
C. The onset of congestive heart failure is associated with an average survival of 3 years
D. The obstruction tends to progress more rapidly in patients with congenital or rheumatic disease than those with degenerative calcific disease
E. The risk of infective endocarditis is higher in older patients with degenerated calcified valves than in younger patients with mild valvular deformity

T T F F F

A large 'a' wave occurs due to a combination of vigorous contraction of a hypertrophic left atrium and reduced LV compliance. A reduced diastolic transmyocardial coronary perfusion gradient is present due to elevated LVEDP and, the sub-endocardium therefore is susceptible to underperfusion. The onset of congestive heart failure is associated with an average survival of 1-1.5 years. Degenerative calcific disease progresses more rapidly.

113

Epidemiologically the risk of endocarditis is higher in younger patients with mild deformity.

Q69 In Hypoplastic Left Heart Syndrome

A. The right ventricle pumps the blood into the pulmonary artery
B. Blood returning from the lungs flows left to right through an atrial septal defect
C. The Norwood procedure is used as a first stage operation to allow the right ventricle to pump blood to both the lungs and the body
D. The Norwood procedure must be performed by three months of age
E. Supplemental oxygen should be commenced at birth

T T T F F

The right ventricle pumps the blood into the pulmonary artery. Blood returning from the lungs flows left to right through an atrial septal defect and admixes with the venous return to the heart and blood reaches the aorta through a patent ductus arteriosus. The Norwood procedure must be performed soon after birth. Supplemental oxygen is avoided as it promotes pulmonary blood flow and may steal blood from the systemic circulation, thus placing further demand on the already stressed right (single) ventricle.

Q70 Regarding concomitant carotid and coronary disease

A. The stroke risk for CEA followed by CABG is superior to alternative strategies
B. CEA followed by CABG has a stroke rate of 1.5 to 3 %

C. Performing CABG and CEA at the same operation has a stroke rate of 3 to 6%
D. The incidences of carotid artery disease is higher in patients who have left main stem coronary disease
E. Carotid stenosis is an independent risk factor of post-CABG stroke

T T T T T

The stroke rates are those observed in the meatanalysis by Das et al (Int J Cardiol 2000; 74: 47–65.) and in the meta-analysis by Borger et al. (Ann Thorac Surg 1999; 68: 14–21.). Individual studies have found perioperative stroke rates up to 9% for combined CEA and CABG. The incidences of carotid artery disease and postoperative cerebrovascular complications is higher in patients who undergo a cardiac revascularisation procedure for stenosis of the left main stem coronary artery.

Q71 Which of the following are true regarding a sinus of Valsalva aneurysm?

A. The majority originate from the right sinus of Valsalva
B. When congenital it is caused by a dilation of a single sinus of Valsalva due to separation between the aortic media and the annulus fibrosus
C. When congenital are associated frequently with atrial septal defects
D. Rupture leading to intracardiac shunting occurs mostly into the right atrium
E. It is best delineated by transthoracic echocardiography

T T F F T

Approximately 75% originate from the right sinus of Valsalva, 20% from the non-coronary sinus, and 5% from the left sinus. Congenital sinus of Valsalva aneurysms are associated with ventricular septal defects. Rupture leading to intracardiac shunting occurs mostly into the right ventricle ($\approx$90%), but may also occur into the right atrium when it is known as a Gerbode defect ($\approx$10%). Cardiac tamponade may occur if the rupture involves the pericardial space. Whilst transthoracic echocardiography may detect as many as 75% often MRI is the most useful diagnostic tool.

Q72 Which of the following are true regarding Rheumatic fever?

A. It develops following pharyngitis with group A beta-haemolytic streptococcus
B. It usually results in constrictive pericarditis
C. The diagnosis of rheumatic fever requires the Dukes criteria
D. Polyarthritis is the most common symptom
E. Streptococcal antigens have structural similarity to laminin in heart valves

T F F T T

Rheumatic fever develops in children and adolescents following pharyngitis with group A beta-haemolytic Streptococcus (Streptococcus pyogenes). The diagnosis of rheumatic fever requires the Jones criteria with the presence of 2 major or 1 major and 2 minor criteria.

Q73 Which statements are true regarding the indications for coronary artery bypass grafting (CABG)?

A. The Veterans' administrative study indicated that CABG was indicated in patients with a ≥50% occlusion of their left main stem coronary artery

B. The Veteran's administrative study indicated that CABG was indicated in patients with proximal triple vessel disease

C. The European Coronary Surgery Study indicated that CABG was indicated in patients with proximal triple vessel disease

D. The Coronary Artery Surgery Study indicated that CABG was indicated in patients with two vessel disease including proximal left anterior descending disease

E. The Coronary Artery Surgery Study indicated that CABG was indicated in patients with impaired ventricular function and triple vessel disease

T T T F T

It was the European Coronary Surgery Study which indicated that CABG was indicated in patients with two vessel disease including proximal left anterior descending disease.

Q74 Which of the following are true of left atrial thrombus?

A. It is rare in the presence of sinus rhythm

B. Thrombus formation is a risk associated with left atrial ablation procedures

C. High plasma homocysteine is an independent risk factor for left atrial thrombus formation in patients with stroke caused by non-valvular atrial fibrillation

D. The presence of spontaneous echo contrast is an independent risk for thrombus formation

E. It is most commonly detected within the left atrial appendage

T T T T T

Homocysteine has been linked to a variety of vascular diseases. Other than being associated with left atrial thrombi large case-control and prospective studies have shown that elevated homocysteine levels are an independent risk factor for arterial and venous thrombotic events. Thrombus is detected within the left atrial appendage in approximately 75% of instances.

Q75 Regarding off pump coronary surgery

    A. An O_2 blower is crucial for beating heart surgery to aid visualisation

    B. Intracoronary shunts are useful in improving haemodynamic stability

    C. Opening the right pleural space facilitates grafting the lateral left ventricular wall

    D. Transoesophageal echocardiography is a better aid to the early detection of myocardial ischemia than ST segment trend monitoring

    E. It may be particularly difficult in patients with severe pectus excavatum

F T T F T

A CO_2 blower is crucial for beating heart surgery at a flow rate adequate for visualisation but not too high to cause damage to the coronary endothelium. The use of CO_2 is important to prevent gas embolisation. Intracoronary shunts are useful in minimising the amount of ischaemia and improving haemodynamic stability. Opening the right pleural space by extending the right pericardial incision towards the inferior vena cava allows the heart to move toward the right beneath the right half of the sternum facilitating access to the lateral left ventricular wall. While transoesophageal echocardiography rapidly demonstrates regional wall motion abnormality, correlating it to regional wall ischaemia is complex due to displacement of the heart and the use of stabilisers. Rightward displacement of the heart may be particularly difficult in patients with severe pectus excavatum.

Q76 Pulmonary artery banding

A. Is performed to prevent irreversible pulmonary hypertension developing
B. Is performed to "train" the left ventricle
C. Is contraindicated in the presence of multiple muscular ventricular septal defects
D. Performed distally is more likely to impinge on the left pulmonary artery than the right
E. Aims to produce a distal pulmonary artery pressure that is a third to half that of systemic pressure

T T F F T

It is performed to reduce excessive pulmonary blood flow and prevent irreversible pulmonary hypertension developing, and also to "train" the left ventricle in patients with transposition of the great arteries having a delayed arterial switch procedure. Multiple muscular ventricular septal defects may be technically difficult to repair in the neonate, and require palliative pulmonary banding until the child is large enough to undertake a corrective procedure. As the right pulmonary artery arises more proximally and also at a more acute angle than the left off the main pulmonary artery it is more susceptible to be impinged upon by a distally placed band.

Q77 Which of the following are true regarding the use of the ACT for assessing anticoagulation for cardiopulmonary bypass?

A. Aprotinin prolongs celite-based ACTs but generally not kaolin-based ACTs
B. The ACT is influenced by haemodilution
C. The ACT measures the activation of the extrinsic pathway of coagulation
D. The ACT is a reliable indication of anticoagulation in a patient undergoing valvular surgery for aortic regurgitation associated with Liebmann Sacks endocarditis
E. The target ACT may vary depending on the test method

T T F F T

When using the ACT, whole blood is collected into a tube containing an activator of coagulation, such as celite (diatomaceous earth), kaolin, or glass particles. These activate the intrinsic pathway of coagulation, causing the blood to clot. The ACT is influenced by lupus anticoagulants that may be present in Liebman Sacks endocarditis of SLE. Hemochron® ACT measurements tend to be higher than HemoTec® ACT measurements, although this is not always the case.

Q78 Which of the following are true regarding cardioplegia?

A. Crystalloid cardioplegic solutions of the intracellular type have absent or low concentrations of sodium and calcium
B. Crystalloid cardioplegic solutions of the extracellular type have higher concentrations of sodium, calcium, and magnesium
C. Crystalloid cardioplegic solutions contain concentrations of potassium greater than 40 mmolL^{-1}
D. Blood cardioplegia provides intermittent re-oxygenation of the arrested heart

E. Cardioplegia solutions used in the paediatric population have lower calcium levels than comparable solutions in adults

T T F T T

In crystalloid cardioplegic solutions the concentration of potassium ranges between 10 mmolL^{-1} and 40 mmolL^{-1}. The calcium metabolism in the paediatric heart is immature and low calcium cardioplegia is used in this age group.

Q79 Which of the following are causes of a continuous cardiac murmur?

A. A patent ductus arteriosus
B. An arterio-venous malformation
C. An aortic root-right atrial fistula
D. A ventricular septal defect
E. A DKS shunt

T T T F T

A continuous cardiac murmur is a heart murmur that occurs throughout the cardiac cycle. This implies flow during both systole and diastole. The murmur may actually be cardiac or non-cardiac in origin. A continuous murmur may be caused by a patent ductus arteriosus, a pulmonary arterio-venous fistula, an intercostal arterio-venous fistula (as may occur following trauma), a ruptured sinus of valsalva aneurysm, coarctation of aorta, a venous hum and a mammary soufflé.

Q80 Rhabdomyoma of the heart

   A. Most commonly occurs in the interventricular septum

   B. Is associated with tuberous sclerosis

   C. Is the most common benign congenital tumour of the heart

   D. On histology shows characteristic spider cells

   E. Requires surgical excision as it is likely to eventually cause haemodynamic compromise even if asymptomatic at detection

T T T T F

The characteristic spider cells are large clear cells with cytoplasmic strands composed of glycogen extending to the plasma membrane. Conservative neonatal management is indicated in the asymptomatic patient as rhabdomyoma cells lose there ability to divide over time, which may account for their spontaneous regression. Surgery is reserved for when there is haemodynamic compromise.

Q81 Which of the following are correct regarding cardiac contusions?

   A. They are most often caused by blunt cardiac injury caused by road traffic accidents

   B. Thay affect the left ventricle more often than the right ventricle

   C. They are histologically characterised by necrosis of myocardial muscle cells

   D. A cardiac contusion is indicated by the elevation of Troponin C

   E. The ECG/EKG is characterised by ST segment or T wave abnormalities

T F T F F

Because of its anterior position and proximity to the sternum, the right ventricle is more frequently injured than the left. Troponin C is also found in skeletal muscles and hence is not specific. In contrast troponin I and troponin T, are highly specific to myocardial injury as they are not found in skeletal muscles and are released into the circulation only after loss of membrane integrity. As the ECG/EKG is relatively insensitive to right ventricular electrical activity most minor cardiac contusions may show none or only minor electrical changes.

'Q82 Which of the following are true of artificial pacing of the heart?

A. Output is measured in millivolts
B. The sensitivity setting is measured in millivolts
C. In a patient who has just arrived on the intensive care unit after cardiac surgery, a pacer spike without a corresponding P wave or QRS complex suggests that the epicardial leads have been dislodged
D. Inappropriate sensing is managed by increasing the sensitivity threshold
E. In type II second-degree AV block with a wide QRS complex, pacing is a Class I recommendation

F T F T T

Output is measured in milliamperes. The sensitivity setting is measured in millivolts and is initially set at about 2 to 5 mV. If the pacemaker is detecting beats that are not actually occurring (inappropriate sensing), then the sensitivity threshold must be increased to block out artifact. A pacer spike without a corresponding P wave or QRS complex indicates failure to capture. If the leads are truly dislodged a pacer spike is unlikely to be seen. A wide QRS complex in patients with type II second-degree AV block suggests diffuse conduction system disease and is considered an indication for pacing even in asymptomatic patients.

Q83 Regarding thoraco-abdominal aortic aneurysms

A. They are most commonly seen in elderly male smokers
B. In the Crawford classification a Type I aneurysm extends into the infra-renal aorta
C. The risk of spinal cord ischaemia is less likely with a type IV thoraco-abdominal aortic aneurysm
D. The "inclusion technique" of repair requires extracorporeal circulation
E. Combined distal aortic perfusion and cerebrospinal fluid drainage improve neurological outcome in repair of thoraco-abdominal aortic aneurysms

T F T F T

In the Crawford classification a Type I aneurysm begins near the left subclavian artery, and extends down to encompose the aorta at the origins of the coeliac axis and superior mesenteric arteries and although the renal arteries may also be involved, the aneurysm does not extend into the infra-renal segment. The "inclusion technique" of repair involves the use of a clamp-and-sew aortic repair with inclusion of the visceral and right renal arteries into the body of the replacement graft as an island of vessels. A graft-to-left renal artery bypass then completes the procedure, all of which was done without extracorporeal circulation. Controlling both the arterial pressure and cerebrospinal fluid (CSF) pressure is critical in preventing spinal cord sequelae and a catheter is inserted into the spinal canal after induction of anaesthesia to maintain CSF pressures ≤10 mm Hg to prevent impedance of spinal cord perfusion.

Q84 Regarding interventional procedures for congenital heart defects

A. Late onset dysrhythmias are more likely to develop following the Mustard procedure than with the Senning procedure

B. The pulmonary arteries must retain the degree of resistance present at birth for the Fontan operation to be successful
C. The modified BT shunt has a propensity to cause excessive pulmonary blood flow
D. A bidirectional Glenn shunt involves connection of the superior and inferior vena cavae to the right PA
E. Pulmonary artery stenosis following surgical repair refractory to balloon dilatation is a contraindication to stenting

T F F F F

The pulmonary arteries must grow well without stenosis and must be of low resistance to allow blood to flow into them without a pump for the Fontan operation to be successful. The main advantages of a modified BT shunt is the limited subclavian artery diameter preventing excessive blood flow, hence, congestive cardiac failure is less likely then with larger shunts such as the Waterston shunt. On the other hand a disadvantage is thrombosis of the shunt due to its small diameter. In a bidirectional Glenn shunt the superior vena cava is connected to the right PA, which is still kept in continuity with the main pulmonary artery allowing blood to flow bidirectionally into both main pulmonary arteries. Stenting has been performed successfully and should be considered in patients with residual or resistant stenosis.

Q85 The following are correct regarding the additive EuroSCORE

A. Being female scores 1 point
B. A 73 year old patient has 2 points added for age
C. Unilateral carotid stenosis of 45% adds 2 points to the score
D. Pulmonary hypertension with Systolic PA pressure>60 mmHg adds 1 point to the score
E. The presence of a post-infarction septal rupture is the single highest scoring risk factor

T F F F T

A point is added for every 5 years or part thereof over 60 years of age. Carotid occlusion or >50% stenosis adds 2 points. Pulmonary hypertension with Systolic PA pressure>60 mmHg adds 2 points to the score. The presence of a post-infarction sepal rupture adds 4 points to the score. The EuroSCORE points system is detailed fully on the official website, which is http://www.euroscore.org/euroscore_scoring.htm

Q86 Systolic anterior motion of the mitral valve

    A. Is explained by a Venturi effect acting on the anterior mitral valve leaflet
    B. Is associated with primary abnormalities of the mitral apparatus
    C. Does not occur before aortic valve opening
    D. Is sensitive to changes in ventricular volume
    E. May be decreased in mitral valve repair by transfer of more posterior leaflet chordae to the anterior leaflet

T T F T T

Systolic anterior motion of the mitral valve is explained by a Venturi effect acting on the anterior mitral valve leaflet related to septal hypertrophy, which causes an outflow tract narrowing and high velocities. These patients also have primary abnormalities of the mitral apparatus, including anterior and inward or central displacement of the papillary muscles, and leaflet elongation, but their relative primary contribution to the causality is open to dabate. The onset of systolic anterior motion of the mitral valve at or before aortic valve opening, when outflow velocity is low has been demonstrated and questions the validity of the venturi effect in this specific setting. Volume replacement may reduce the degree of impingement into the left ventricular outflow tract.

Posteriorly directed posterior leaflet secondary chordae may be transferred to the underside of the mid-anterior leaflet to draw the anterior leaflet away from the left ventricular outflow tract at the time of mitral valve repair.

Q87 Indications for thrombolytic therapy after an acute myocardial infarction include which of the following?

A. ST segment elevation (> 0.1 mV)
B. ST segment depression
C. New left bundle branch block
D. Presentation within 12 hours of the onset of symptoms
E. Coronary ischaemia associated with a type A aortic dissection

T F T T F

ST segment depression is not generally considered an indication unless anterior ST depression is considered to be due to a posterior infarction. Although used within the first 12 hours of an MI, effectiveness is greatest in the first 2 hours and rapidly decreases thereafter.

Q88 Which of the following are true of protein loosing enteropathy?

A. It is associated with hypoalbuminaemia.
B. It is characterised by the absence of α1-antitrypsin in the stools
C. The diets of patients should be supplemented with fat-soluble vitamins A, D, E, and K
D. When occurring after a Fontan procedure, fenestration of the baffle separating the systemic venous from the pulmonary venous pathway should be performed

E. Cardiac transplantation should be considered if associated with a previous fenestrated Fontan operation

T F T T T

Protein loosing enteropathy is characterised by the presence of α1-antitrypsin in the stools.

✓ Q89 Which of the following regarding left ventricular aneurysms are correct?

A. They are associated with an abnormal precordial impulse
B. They are associated with persistent elevation of the S-T segment on ECG/EKG
C. Medical treatment with spironolactone improves survival
D. Echocardiography is unable to differentiate between true and false aneurysms
E. Mural thrombi are present in about half of all left ventricular aneurysms

T T T F T

A quarter of patients with a ventricular aneurysm show persistent ST elevation in the territory of the myocardial infarction. A dominant R wave in lead aVF may also be a helpful pointer. Medical treatment has been shown to extend 50% survival to 6.5 years (ACE inhibitors), 7.5 years (β-blockers) and 8.5 years (spironolactone). The differentiation between true and false aneurysms is aided by echocardiography, with true left ventricular aneurysms having a wide mouth while false aneurysms often extend behind the intact left ventricular wall and have a narrow neck.

Q90 Which of the following are true regarding atrial isomerism?

    A. Bilateral bilobar lungs with 'long bronchi' are associated with right atrial isomerism

    B. Bilateral trilobar lungs with 'short bronchi' are associated with right atrial isomerism

    C. A dual sinus node or dual AV node is associated with left atrial isomerism

    D. Absent sinus node and complete heart block is associated with left atrial isomerism

    E. Polysplenism is associated with left atrial isomerism

F T F T T

Bilateral bilobar lungs with 'long bronchi' are associated with left atrial isomerism. A dual sinus node or dual AV node is associated with right atrial isomerism.

Q91 Which of the following are true regarding a pericardial effusion?

    A. The classic Beck triad of pericardial tamponade consists of hypotension, muffled heart sounds, and jugular venous distension

    B. It may be associated with a pulsus paradoxus

    C. It is not differentiated from a pleural effusion by echocardiography

    D. The initial treatment of tuberculous pericarditis includes the use of antituberculous drugs and prednisolone

    E. It is differentiated from a viral cardiomyopathy by echocardiography

T T F T T

A pulsus paradoxus is a decrease in systolic blood pressure of more than 10 mm Hg with inspiration. False-positive echocardiographic diagnosis can occur in pleural effusions, pericardial thickening, and increased pericardial fat as well as with cystic mediastinal lesions. Nonetheless the descending aorta may be used as a marker to differentiate a pericardial effusion from a pleural effusion. Although the role of adjunctive corticosteroids in reducing mortality or progression to constriction in tuberculous pericarditis exists it tends to be used in the first 4-6 weeks of treatment, especially in the acute setting. A viral cardiomyopathy may have a similar presentation, with an enlarged heart on chest radiographs. Echocardiography readily distinguishes between enlarged cardiac chambers associated with viral cardiomyopathy, and a pericardial effusion.

'Q92 Regarding conventional coronary angiography

A. A 6F catheter used in coronary angiography has an outer diameter of 2 mm
B. In the LAO view the vertebral column is visualised on the left of the image
C. It is associated with elevations in interleukin-6 levels
D. The angiographic severity of coronary stenosis accurately predicts the location of a subsequent coronary occlusion that will produce a myocardial infarction
E. It is inferior to electron beam CT coronary angiography for the distal coronary circulation

T T T F F

Cardiac catheters are referred to in "French" units equivalent to the outer diameters, with one "French" unit being 0.33 mm. In patients undergoing coronary interventions, striking elevations in interleukin-6 levels (as much as 9- and 13-fold increases in angiography and PCI respectively) have been observed. The literature suggests that assessment of the angiographic severity of coronary stenosis is inadequate to accurately predict the time or location of a subsequent coronary occlusion that will produce a myocardial infarction. Approximately 20% of coronary artery segments are un-analysable by electron beam CT coronary angiography. The location of these un-analysable segments is proximal in 8%, middle in 22% and distal in 70%.

Q93 Regarding aortic root enlargement

A. The Konno-Rastan procedure is a posterior enlargement of the aortic root
B. The Konno-Rastan procedure may damage the first septal artery
C. The Nicks procedure involves extending the aortotomy through the posterior commissure into the interleaflet triangle
D. Posterior aortic root enlargement techniques can be used without additional operative risk
E. The Manouguian's Technique enlarges the root through the non-coronary annulus

F T T T T

The Konno-Rastan procedure is an anterior enlargement where the incision of the infundibular septum can result in division of the first septal artery. Unlike anterior enlargement posterior enlargement, can be achieved without additional operative risk, especially with more limited enlargement to upsize by 2 - 4 mm.

Q94 Which of the following are correct regarding the Norwood operation?

A. It converts the morphologic right ventricle into the systemic ventricle
B. It is a means of palliating conditions in which the morphologic left ventricle is inadequate in maintaining systemic circulation
C. It uses the pulmonary artery to construct a neo-aorta
D. It involves creating a Glenn shunt
E. It uses α blockade with phenoxybenzamine in the postoperative management

T T F T T

The Norwood operation involves creating a Blalock-Tausig shunt. A Glenn shunt is inappropriate in this first stage palliative procedure performed early after birth when the pulmonary vascular resistance is still high. The principle of using α blockade is the increase in systemic cardiac output that occurs due to maximal dilatation of the systemic circulation. This effect results in a more stable parallel circulation through prevention of fluctuations in systemic vascular resistance in the early postoperative period.

Q95 Which of the following are true regarding atrial flutter?

A. Type I flutter is called typical flutter
B. With type I atrial flutter, directionality around the tricuspid valve annulus is invariably clockwise
C. Type II atrial flutter often result from previous surgical atriotomy scars
D. It is not a cause of left atrial thrombus
E. The likelihood of cure for patients with Type I atrial flutter who undergo catheter ablation is poor

T F T F F

With type I atrial flutter, directionality around the tricuspid valve annulus can be clockwise (uncommon) or counter clockwise (common). Type II atrial flutter does not require the tricuspid annular isthmus for a re-entrant circuit and often results from previous surgical scars of the atrium. Thrombus in the left atrium has been described with thromboembolic complications. The prognosis for patients with Type I atrial flutter who undergo catheter ablation is good.

Q96 Regarding myocardial perfusion imaging

A. Adenosine stress testing is unreliable in a patient who has had a cup of coffee on the way for the test
B. A fixed anterior wall defect is indicative of an unviable old infarction
C. Thallium is taken up by viable myocytes and is proportional to coronary blood flow
D. Technicium 99m sestamibi is less useful to identify viable myocardium than Thallium 201
E. PET is useful for distinguishing idiopathic from ischaemic dilated cardiomyopathy

T F T T T

If a pharmacologic stress test with a vasodilator such as adenosine or dipyridamole is to be performed caffeine should be avoided for 12 to 24 hours as it blocks adenosine receptors on arterial smooth muscle cells. A fixed perfusion defect along the anterior wall of the LV could well be due to breast attenuation, especially if associated with normal motion and thickening on the gated study. Technicium 99m sestamibi is a calcium analogue that undergoes minimal myocardial redistribution (uptake) and hence is less useful for viability studies. In a PET scan patchy perfusion defects (decreased tracer uptake) with an enlarged left ventricle is indicative of ischaemic dilated cardiomyopathy, since there is a low flow state (ischaemia) and dilatation of the myocardium. If the FDG metabolic study is normal, revascularisation is a potential management approach. If the metabolism study shows a low metabolic state, revascularisation would be of little benefit.

Q97 Which of the following are correct regarding exercise ECG testing?

A. Horizontal or downsloping ST segment depression of 0.1 mV or more for 80 ms is a poitive test
B. ST segment elevation in patients with no Q waves on the resting ECG is a positive test
C. Patients with complete left bundle branch block are preferably tested with an imaging modality rather than with exercise ECG testing
D. ST segment elevation may occur over a ventricular aneurysm during exercise ECG testing
E. A normal ECG during exercise testing excludes the risk of ischaemic heart disease

T T T T F

Patients with left bundle branch block should usually be tested with an imaging modality but exercise testing may still provide prognostic information such as exercise capacity although it cannot be used to identify ischaemia. ST segment elevation may occur over dyskinetic areas.

Q98 Regarding the history of cardiac surgery

A. Shumway and Lower are credited for first using hypothermic techniques to protect the heart during ischaemic periods
B. Bretschneider developed buffering techniques for cardioplegia solutions
C. HS Suttar is the first documented to have successfully performed a mitral valvulotomy
D. Donald Ross performed the first successful aortic valve replacement with an aortic valve homograft
E. Carpentier performed the first successful xenograft valve replacement

T T F T T

HS Suttar is the first documented to have successfully performed a mitral valvotomy using his finger to fracture the commissures, as surgical treatment of mitral stenosis. Elliott Cutler is considered the first to have performed a surgical valvotomy a few years prior to that.

Q99 Which of the following are true regarding studies on coronary revascularisation?

A. The ECSS demonstrated a significant survival advantage for surgery when compared to medical therapy alone at 5 years follow up
B. The RITA study showed a greater need for repeat revascularisation in patients receiving angioplasty than those receiving surgery
C. The ARTS study compared isolated ballon angioplasty to surgery
D. The SoS trial compared coronary stenting with surgery

E. The AWESOME trial found a significant 5 year survival advantage for stenting as compared to surgery in high risk patients

T T F T F

The ARTS study compared coronary stenting with surgery. The AWESOME trial found no significant difference in mortality at 5 years, symptom free status, myocardial infarction or revascularisation, between stenting and surgery in high risk patients.

✓Q100 Which of the following are correct of aortic regurgitation?

A. It is associated with ankylosing spondilitis
B. When acute it is associated with closure of the mitral valve in diastole
C. It is associated with a soft mid-diastolic rumble heard at the apical area
D. The regurgitation is considered severe if the pressure half time is >250 ms
E. When due to aortic valve endocarditis, valve replacement should be delayed for at least 4-6 weeks

T T T F F

In acute regurgitation since the left ventricle has not yet developed eccentric hypertrophy and dilatation, the elevated filling pressures can close the mitral valve early. An Austin Flint murmur, a soft mid-diastolic rumble heard at the apical area occurs when the regurgitant jet causes closure of the anterior mitral leaflet. It is severe if the pressure half time is <250 ms. In regurgitant conditions the shorter the pressure half time the more severe the condition.

CHAPTER 3

Thoracic Surgery

Q1 Which of the following details regarding the Masaoka staging system for thymoma are correct?

   A. Stage I thymoma is limited to the thymus without invasion of its capsule

   B. Stage IIa thymoma has microscopic invasion into the capsule

   C. Stage IIb thymoma has macroscopic invasion into surrounding fatty tissue or mediastinal pleura

   D. Stage III thymoma grossly invades lung, pericardium or the great vessels

   E. Stage IVb thymoma has extrathoracic metastases

T F F T T

	The Masaoka Staging System for Thymoma
Stage	Description
I	Macroscopically completely encapsulated, microscopically no capsular invasion
IIa	Macroscopic invasion into surrounding fatty tissue or mediastinal pleura
IIb	Microscopic invasion into capsule
III	Macroscopic invasion into neighbouring organs (pericardium, lung, and great vessels)
IVa	Pleural or pericardial dissemination
IVb	Lymphatogenous or haematogenous metastases outside thorax

Q2 Which of the following are true of tracheal tumours?

A. The vast majority of tracheal tumours are malignant
B. Adenoid cystic carcinoma is evenly distributed between males and females
C. Ectopic thyroid tissue within the trachea should be managed conservatively by annual bronchoscopy
D. Squamous papillomas are the commonest of the benign tracheal tumours
E. Cartilaginous tumours if not obstructive do not require surgical intervention

T T F T F

Thyroid tissue may be present ectopically within the trachea and should be excised as it has the potential for malignant change. Squamous papillomas are the commonest of the benign tracheal tumours and are associated with human papilloma virus types 6 and 11. Cartilaginous tumours may undergo sarcomatous change and should be excised where possible.

Q3 Which of the following are true of cryptococcal lung infection?

A. It commonly manifests as a cavitating lung lesion
B. It is a cause of ARDS in immunocompromised individuals
C. It is characterised by hilar lymphadenopathy
D. It causes granulomatous and miliary disease similar to pulmonary tuberculosis
E. It is transmitted by organ transplantation

F T F T T

C neoformans, an encapsulated yeast, causes the vast majority of cryptococcal infections in patients who are immunosuppressed. Cavitation and hilar lymphadenopathy are infrequent. Radiographic findings including patchy pneumonitis, granulomas, or miliary disease similar to tuberculosis may occur in immunocompetent patients.

Q4 Which of the following regarding lung transplantation are true?

A. Lung transplantation should be offered to patients with emphysema who have an FEV_1 substantially less than 30% predicted
B. Severe restrictive disease, hypoxaemia, and poor performance status are criteria used for transplant consideration
C. In patients with primary pulmonary hypertension and NYHA class III and IV symptoms transplant is indicated only if the patients cannot tolerate or fail prostacyclin therapy
D. Current corticosteroid treatment is a contraindication to transplantation
E. Patients with cystic fibrosis require bilateral lung transplantation

T T T F T

An FEV_1 of less than 30% predicted is associated with a 60-80% 2-year survival rate. An FVC of less than 67% predicted is associated with an approximately 50% survival rate at 2 years. Although there are concerns about anastomotic dehiscence, low-dose steroid therapy (i.e. <20 mg/d) may be acceptable.

Q5 Which of the following are true regarding infections in lung transplant recipient patients?

A. Non-tuberculous mycobacterial colonisation is considered a contraindication to lung transplantation
B. Aspergillus fumigatus colonisation of a patient with cystic fibrosis is only a relative contraindication
C. The presence of infection with B cepacia in patients with cystic fibrosis, is associated with significant mortality rates
D. Cytomegalovirus infections are eliminated by routine acyclovir prophylaxis after lung transplantation
E. Pneumocystis carinii infection can be eliminated by the routine use of trimethoprim-sulfamethoxazole

F T T F T

Some centres do not offer transplants to patients infected with B cepacia. Cytomegalovirus infections are eliminated by routine gancyclovir.

Q6 The 1994 American-European Consensus Committee definition of ARDS (acute respiratory distress syndrome) incorporates the following

A. The acute onset of bilateral infiltrates on chest radiography
B. A partial pressure of arterial oxygen (PaO_2) to fraction of inspired oxygen (F_iO_2) ratio of less than 200 mm Hg
C. A pulmonary artery occlusion pressure of less than 18
D. The absence of clinical evidence of elevated left arterial pressure
E. It should not occur in the context of cardiac surgery

T T T T F

It is distinguished from acute lung injury, which is similar to ARDS with the exception of a PaO_2/F_IO_2 ratio of less than 300 mm Hg. ARDS has been associated with protamine administration and also with multiple blood transfusions in the setting of cardiac surgery.

Q7 The following are features of the acute respiratory distress syndrome

A. It results from damage to the alveolar epithelium and vascular endothelium leading to the passage of plasma and inflammatory cells into the interstitium and alveolar space
B. The presence of a third heart sound (S_3) on auscultation of the heart is a feature of the condition
C. A decreased alveolar-arterial oxygen gradient occurs
D. It may lead to fibrosing alveolitis within the first week
E. Its management includes stringently keeping the PCO_2 within the normal range

T F F T F

Signs of volume overload, such as an S_3 on auscultation of the heart should be absent. An increased alveolar-arterial oxygen gradient occurs. Management involves using lower tidal volumes and allowing hypercapnia (permissive hypercapnia) to develop if peak airway pressures rise.

Q8 Which of the following are true of lymphangioleiomyomatosis?

A. It is a disease of postmenopausal women
B. It is a cause of chylothorax
C. It characteristically shows a fine nodular pattern on high resolution CT scanning

D. Pulmonary function tests show a decreased diffusing capacity for carbon monoxide
E. It is an indication for lung transplantation

F T F T T

It typically occurs in premenopausal women and hence involvement of the female hormones in disease pathogenesis is hypothesised. Proliferation of neoplastic cells with smooth muscle cell phenotypia (LAM cell) occurs in the lung, kidney, and axial lymphatics, causing obstructive pathology. High resolution CT scanning characteristically shows diffuse thin-walled cysts. Lung transplantation should be considered for patients with end-stage pulmonary disease.

Q9 Which of the following are correct regarding tracheobronchial rupture?

A. It occurs less often with blunt trauma than with penetrating injuries
B. When oral intubation is not satisfactory jet ventilation through intra-bronchial catheters, inserted via emergency thoracotomy, should be used
C. An elevated PCO_2 at the time of admission is associated with a poorer prognosis
D. A patch repair may be performed using an intercostal muscle flap
E. It can be treated with antibiotics and intubation with the cuff inflated proximal to the tear

F T T T F

The use of an on-lay patch reduces the likelihood of stenosis at the site. Localised short lacerations, especially if they do not involve the whole thickness of the tracheal wall, can be treated with antibiotics and intubation with the cuff inflated distal to the tear, and avoiding high ventilation pressures.

Q10 Which of the following conditions is associated with an increased incidence of adenocarcinoma of the oesophagus?

A. Tylosis
B. Barrett's oesophagus
C. Oesophageal strictures
D. Plummer-Vinson syndrome
E. Hiatus hernia

F T F F F

Tylosis and Plummer-Vinson syndrome are associated with an increased incidence of squamous cell carcinoma of the oesophagus. Hiatus hernia does not have an increased association with carcinoma of the oesophagus.

Q11 Which of the following statements regarding adenocarcinoma of the oesophagus are true?

A. The incidence of adenocarcinoma of the oesophagus has increased 300% to 500% in the western world during the last 30 to 40 years
B. The absolute risk of any given patient with Barrett oesophagus developing cancer in a year is approximately 1 in 200
C. Cigarette smoking has been shown to be a significant risk factor
D. Alcohol consumption has been shown to be a significant risk factor

E. Daily intake of 75mg of aspirin has been shown to be a significant risk factor

T T T F F

Alcohol consumption does not appear to increase the risk of adenocarcinoma of the oesophagus, but increases the risk of developing squamous cell carcinoma of the oesophagus. Consumption of wine, aspirin, and the presence of certain strains of H. pylori, may be protective and lessen the risk of oesophageal adenocarcinoma.

Q12 Which of the following are true of myasthenia gravis?

A. There are decreased nicotinic postsynaptic receptors at the myoneural junction
B. Patients become symptomatic once the number of ACh receptors is reduced to approximately 30% of normal
C. Exacerbations may be provoked by β-blockers
D. Patients with ocular symptoms have class III myasthenia gravis
E. Anti-AChR antibodies assays are positive in over 90% of patients with isolated ocular disease

T T T F F

Exacerbations may be provoked by antibiotics, antidysrhythmic agents, muscle relaxants, and paradoxically, corticosteroids. Anti-AChR antibodies are present in 90% of patients with generalized disease but only 50-70% of patients with isolated ocular disease. The modified classification of symptoms is outlined below.

Class I	Ocular
Class II	Mild generalised weakness
Class III	Bulbar disease
Class IV	Moderate generalised weakness
Class V	Severe generalised weakness

Q13 Which of the following regarding thymectomy for myasthenia gravis are correct?

A. A CT scan or MR imaging of the chest and mediastinum is part of the diagnostic evaluation of all patients
B. In myasthenia gravis patients are more likely to be improved or in remission if thymectomy is performed within the first year of the onset of symptoms
C. Overall approximately 50% of patients with myasthenia gravis experience improvement
D. Minimally invasive techniques have equivalent efficacy compared to conventional open techniques
E. A transcervical approach may be used

T T F T T

Approximately 85% of patients with myasthenia gravis experience improvement. Minimally invasive techniques have become increasingly popular due to their low procedural morbidity and mortality, cosmesis, and equivalent efficacy compared to conventional open techniques.

✓Q14 Which of the following are true regarding haemoptysis?

A. In most cases it results from disruption of branches of the bronchial arterial system
B. It may be seen in patients with bronchiectasis
C. Massive haemoptysis is a common complication of tuberculosis
D. When massive the cause of death is hypovolaemia
E. When treated with bronchial artery embolisation, has a late re-bleeding rate of 10-20% due to incomplete embolisation

T T F F F

Massive haemoptysis has been arbitrarily defined as the expectoration of more than 600 mL of blood in 24 hours and most deaths are due to asphyxia and hypoxaemia from aspiration of blood into other areas of the lung. Massive fatal haemoptysis in patients with chronic cavitary tuberculosis can result from rupture of a pulmonary artery aneurysm (Rasmussen's aneurysm) in the walls of a tuberculous cavity, but is rare. Bronchial arterial embolisation is associated with late re-bleeding in 10% to 20% of patients by 1 year due to proliferation of collateral vessels.

Q15 Which of the following are true of cavitating lung disease?

A. It is associated with staphylococcal endocarditis
B. It is unusual in Klebsiella pneumonia
C. When affecting an anterior segment is reason for a strong suspicion of lung cancer
D. Cavities due to Mycobacterium avium intracellulare are characteristically large
E. When associated with Nocardia is often multicavitatory

T F T T T

TB and aspiration lung abscess are rare in anterior segments, lung cancer can occur in any segment.

Q16 Which of the following are causes of cavitatory lung disease where the cavities radiographically appear thick walled?

A. Lung abscess
B. Necrotizing squamous cell lung cancer
C. Metastatic cavitating squamous cell carcinoma from outside the lung
D. Blastomycosis
E. Coccidioidomycosis

T T F T F

Thick walled cavities are also seen in Wegener's granulomatosis. Thin walled caiteis are also seen in M. Kansasii infection, congenital or acquired bullae, with post-traumatic cysts and open inactive TB.

Q17 The following are correct regarding chest wall tumours

A. Fibrous dysplasia is the most common tumour of the ribs
B. A painful expansion on the posterior or lateral aspect of a rib is characteristic of fibrous dysplasia
C. Chondrosarcoma is the most common primary malignant tumour of the entire chest wall
D. Histological grade relates poorly to the outcome in patients with a chest wall chondrosarcoma
E. Most chest wall tumours found in children are primary, while most found in adults are secondary

T F T F T

147

Benign tumours of the chest wall are not uncommon. Cancerous tumours, on the other hand, are rare and account for only 5% of all thoracic malignancies.

Q18 Which of the following are correct regarding chylothorax?

A. It is confirmed by a triglyceride level of 110 mg/dl or greater
B. It is associated with leucopoenia and malnutrition
C. Meta analysis of studies shows that the use of somatostatin significantly reduces the quantity and duration of the condition
D. In a left chylothorax associated with an Ivor Lewis operation re-operation is best performed through the left hemithorax
E. Percutaneous thoracic duct catheterisation and embolisation is performed in patients who have lymphangioleiomyomatosis associated chylothorax

T T F F F

In a left chylothorax associated with an Ivor Lewis operation re-operation is best performed through the right hemithorax as the patient does not have to recover from bilateral thoracotomies and a pleurodesis can be used to obliterate the pleural space as the duct lies on the right side in most of its course. Percutaneous thoracic duct catheterisation and embolisation has been successfully performed in patients with patent major retroperitoneal lymphatic trunks, but lymphangioleiomyomatosis can lead to silent occlusion of these trunks and hence a significant failure rate.

Q19 Regarding pulmonary thromboembolism

A. The average mortality rate is 10 to 15%
B. Calf vein deep vein thrombosis does not cause pulmonary embolism
C. The most frequent symptoms and signs of PE are non specific
D. The PaO$_2$ on arterial blood gases analysis is predictive of the likelihood of a pulmonary embolus
E. A high white blood cell count makes the diagnosis unlikely

T F T F F

Approximately 10% of patients in whom acute PE is diagnosed die. The most frequent symptom and signs of PE are non specific, such as dyspnoea, tachypnoea, tachycardia and chest pain. They can be found in other clinical situations. The PO$_2$ on arterial blood gase analysis has no predictive value in a typical population of patients. The white blood cell count may be normal or elevated and a high count is not uncommon in patients with pulmonary thromboembolism.

Q20 Which of the following are true of dysplasia of the oesophagus?

A. It is also known as Barrett's oesophagus
B. The cell nucleus to cytoplasm ratio is increased
C. Loss of mitotic figures occurs
D. Depletion of mucin is a feature
E. If confirmed it requires oesophagectomy

F T F T T

Historically Barrett's oesophagus has been differentiated from dysplasia although there is evidence to suggest that non-dysplastic (metaplastic) epithelium in Barrett's oesophagus possesses many of the biological characteristics of "neoplastic" epithelium. Cytologically, regenerating cells contain nuclei with smooth membranes, normal nucleus to cytoplasm ratio, and a variable number of normal mitoses, but may also show prominent nucleoli without significant enlargement. Nuclear pleomorphism, loss of cell polarity and markedly raised nucleus to cytoplasm ratio are features accepted as those of dysplasia. In dysplasia mucin depletion is prominent and goblet cells, both typical and dystrophic, are markedly decreased in number.

Q21 Which of the following types of columnar epithelium may be present in Barrett's oesophagus?

A. Intestinal (Goblet cell) metaplasia
B. Pseudostratified ciliated columnar
C. Gastric cardiac type (junctional)
D. Fundic type
E. Stratified columnar

T F T T F

The term Barrett's oesophagus is used to describe the change from the normal stratified squamous epithelium of the lower oesophagus to a polarised, columnar-lined epithelium with intestinal-type differentiation. This condition develops in the context of chronic gastro-oesophageal reflux disease and is associated with a 0.5–1% annual conversion rate to oesophageal adenocarcinoma.

Q22 Pulmonary alveolar proteinosis

    A. Shows PAS (+) alveolar material derived from surfactant to be present
    B. May be idiopathic
    C. Is associated with lung infection due to Nocardia asteroids
    D. Is seen in inhalation of aluminium oxides
    E. Is a relentlessly progressive condition

T T T T F

Pulmonary alveolar proteinosis is a rare disease in which the alveoli become plugged with a protein-rich fluid. The cause is unknown. Occasionally, it is related to exposure to toxic substances, such as inorganic dusts, infections, cancers and immunosuppressant drugs. The disease may progress, remain stable, or disappear spontaneously.

Q23 Which of the following predispose to spontaneous pneumothorax?

    A. Emphysema
    B. Lymphangiomyomatosis
    C. Bronchiectasis
    D. Fibrosing alveolitis
    E. Oeosinophilic granulomatosis

T T F T T

When pneumothorax occurs without preceding trauma, it is classified as spontaneous pneumothorax, either primary (without clinically or radiographically apparent lung or chest wall disease) or secondary (when such disease is present). The characteristic feature of lymphangiomyomatosis is extensive smooth muscle proliferation involving the pulmonary lymphatics, blood vessels and airways. Muscular hyperplasia of the bronchiolar walls results in luminal narrowing and air trapping, with overdistention of distal air spaces resulting in bullous change and pneumothoraces. Oeosinophilic granulomatosis is histologically characterized by abnormal infiltration of the lungs by Langerhans cells and Spontaneous pneumothorax is a common complication occurring in approximately 10-20% of patients.

Q24 The incidence of cancer of the lung is increased in

A. Cigarette smokers
B. Persons exposed to radon gas
C. Patients with scarring from previous lung disease
D. Persons exposed to nickel
E. Asbestos exposure

T T T T T

The risk of lung cancer in cigarette smokers is related most to the duration of being a smoker. Fifteen years after stopping smoking, the risk of getting lung cancer is almost down to that of a non-smoker. Passive smoking increases the risk of lung cancer and the risk to passive smokers goes up the more cigarette smoke they are exposed to. There is about a 25% increased risk of lung cancer in non-smoking husbands or wives of heavy smokers. Asbestos increases the risk of getting lung cancer, as do uranium, chromium and nickel. Radon gas is a natural gas that can seep out of the soil into buildings. This is more likely in certain parts of the U.K. such as the West Country and Peak District where there is a lot of granite. Radon is considered to be the second leading cause of lung cancer in the U.S.

Q25 The following are true regarding the TNM staging of lung cancer

A. A tumour in the right main bronchus bronchoscopically 1.5cm from the carina is a T4 tumour
B. Satellite nodules within the ipsilateral primary tumour lobe are staged as a T4 tumour
C. A superior sulcus tumour invading the chest wall is a T4 tumour
D. Involvement of ipsilateral paratracheal lymph nodes indicates N3 disease
E. Non-contiguous metastatic tumour nodules in an ipsilateral non-primary lobe is staged as M1 disease

F T F F T

The TNM staging system for lung cancer describes the extent of anatomic involvement by the disease process. This is achieved by defining the characteristics of the primary tumour (T), regional lymph node involvement (N), and metastatic disease (M). It is important for treatment and prognostic reasons. As the classification may undergo periodic revisions readers are advised to familiarise themselves with the latest version.

Q26 Blastomycosis

A. Is a granulomatous fungal condition
B. Is caused by inhalation of aerolised conidial forms that subsequently transform into yeasts
C. Results in asymptomatic pulmonary infection in 25% of patients
D. Is commonly associated with pleural effusions
E. On sputum microscopy shows yeasts with single broad based buds, double refractile walls, and multiple nuclei that are diagnostic

T T F F T

Asymptomatic pulmonary infection occurs in one half of patients.

Q27 Which of the following are correct regarding pneumonia?

A. Bronchopneumonia is more common in infancy and old age
B. Lobar pneumonia is usually due to Strep pneumoniae
C. Red hepatisation in lobar pneumonia is assssociated with infiltration of the alveoli with neutrophils
D. It may be associated with hyponatraemia
E. The mortality for methicillin-resistant Staphylococcus aureus (MRSA) pneumonia in ventilated patients approximates 25%

T T T T F

Hyponatraemia in pneumonia is thought to be due to extra anti-diuretic hormone (SIADH). In red hepatisation both red cell and neutrophil infiltration is seen. The mortality for methicillin-resistant Staphylococcus aureus (MRSA) pneumonia in ventilated patients approximates 50%.

Q28 Which of the following are true of bronchiectasis?

A. It is characterised by irreversible dilatation of the affected bronchus
B. It is associated with cystic fibrosis
C. It may be initiated by the measles virus
D. The presence of bronchi within 1cm of the pleura on high resolution CT scanning is a radiological diagnostic criterion

E. Lung transplantation is reserved for patients with a life expectancy of less than two years and no significant co-morbidity

F T T T T

There are three types of bronchiectasis – 1. Cylindrical, the most common with slight widening of the respiratory passages, can be reversed, and is seen after acute bronchitis. 2. Varicose, where bronchial walls have both extended and collapsed portions like varicosities in veins. 3. Cystic, the most severe, involving irreversible ballooning of the bronchi. On High Resolution Computed Tomography scanning of the lungs the criteria for the diagnosis of bronchiectasis are lack of tapering, visibility of bronchi within 1cm of the pleura and bronchial dilatation.

Q29 Bronchial carcinoid

A. Is a neuro-endocrine tumour originating from bronchial mucosa
B. Is often located in the periphery of the lung
C. May present as recurrent chest infections
D. Has an avidity for octreotide due to the presence of somatostatin receptors
E. Is differentiated from lung cancer in being PET negative

T F T T F

Bronchial carcinoid tumours arise from Kulchitsky cells within the bronchial mucosa. These cells are predominantly distributed proximally at the bifurcation of the lobar bronchi.

Q30 Which of the following are true of bronchial carcinoid?

A. It typically show a marked female predilection
B. It typically metastasises to regional lymph nodes
C. Atypical tumours characteristically affect older males
D. Atypical tumours show osteolytic bony metastases
E. Five-year survival after surgical resection for atypical tumours is 60%

T F T F T

Typical bronchial carcinoid tumours are well defined, small, and central and affect relatively young patients, with a marked female predilection (female-to-male ratio is 10:1), and with endobronchial growth. Atypical carcinoids account for 25% of lung carcinoid tumours, and are more aggressive, affecting older males, tend to occupy a peripheral location, with regional lymph node metastases being more common and occurring in up to 50% of patients. Distant metastases to the liver, bone (osteoblastic), and brain are reported in one third. Five-year survival after surgical resection for typical tumours is >90%.

Q31 Which of the following statements regarding proven aetiological factors and associations of lung cancer are true?

A. Cigarette smoking causes an at least 20 fold increase in likelihood
B. Asbestos exposure causes a multiplicative risk in smokers
C. The Epstein-Barr virus increases the likelihood of squamous cell cancer
D. Interstitial pulmonary fibrosis is a risk factor for its development
E. Radon exposure causes a multiplicative risk in smokers

T T F T T

The effect of asbestos exposure is indeed multiplicative rather than simply additive in cigarette smokers. Exposure to radon in combination with cigarette smoking greatly increases the risk of lung cancer.

Q32 Which of the statements are accurate of emphysema?

A. The pan-acinar type is associated with $\alpha 1$-antitrypsin deficiency
B. The pan-acinar type affects predominantly the lower lobes
C. The centrilobar type is associated with cigarette smoking
D. The centrilobar type affects predominantly the upper lobes
E. It is associated with proliferation of elastin cells

T T T T F

Panacinar emphysema destroys the entire alveolus uniformly and is predominant in the lower half of the lungs. This type of emphysema generally is observed in patients with homozygous $\alpha 1$-antitrypsin deficiency. In people who smoke, focal panacinar emphysema at the lung bases may accompany centriacinar emphysema. Centriacinar emphysema begins in the respiratory bronchioles and spreads peripherally and is also called centrilobular emphysema. It is associated with cigarette smoking and predominantly involves the upper half of the lungs. In a third type known as distal acinar emphysema (paraseptal emphysema), the process is localized around the septae of the lungs or pleura. Although airflow is frequently preserved, apical bullae may lead to spontaneous pneumothorax.

Q33 Which of the following is true regarding sarcoidosis?

A. It is a cause of hilar lympadenopathy
B. Extrarenal vitamin D production can be marked
C. The vital capacity is decreased
D. Minocycline is used in its treatment
E. Elevated levels of ACE differentiate it from granulomatous fungal lung disease

T T T T F

Macrophages within the granulomas convert vitamin D to its active form. It mostly manifests as a restrictive disease but obstructive features can be present due to external compression of airways by lympadenopathy. Cell wall deficient bacteria that are acid fast L forms, have been grown under special conditions from the blood of patients with sarcoidosis, and recently (2006), Minocycline has been designated for use in the treatment of sarcoidosis by the FDA. ACE levels are elevated in sarcoidosis, but also in fungal diseases, HIV, and lymphoma and hence are more useful for monitoring active disease progress in sarcoidosis.

Q34 Which of the following are true of small cell cancer of the lung?

A. It occurs more often in males
B. It shows nuclear moulding on histology
C. Surgical resection of the primary tumour has no role in its management
D. The survival following chemotherapy is worse in patients with superior vena caval obstruction
E. The overall survival at 5 years is 25%

T T F F F

At the time of diagnosis, approximately 1/3 of patients with small cell carcinoma will have tumour confined to the ipsilateral hemithorax, the mediastinum, or the supraclavicular lymph nodes. These patients are designated as having limited-stage disease. A small proportion of patients with early limited-stage disease may benefit from surgery with or without adjuvant chemotherapy. Patients with tumours that have spread beyond the supraclavicular areas are said to have extensive-stage disease and have a worse prognosis. When treated with chemotherapy, the median survival times with or without superior vena caval syndrome are almost identical. The overall survival at 5 years is 5% to 10%.

Q35 Which of the following are correct regarding tuberculosis?

A. Pulmonary infection occurs due to the inhalation of mycobacterial spores
B. It shows highly virulant transmissision
C. It is associated with silicosis
D. Reactivation pulmonary tuberculosis usually ocurs in the upper lobes
E. Calcification related to old tuberculous pericarditis is best seen on MRI scanning.

F F T T T

Pulmonary infection occurs due to the inhalation of bacillus laden droplets. The stringent growth requirements of the organism dictate that it requires a prolonged exposure period.

Q36 Adenocarcinoma of the lung

A. Tends to be peripherally located
B. Is more likely to be associated with a hypercoagulable state than squamous cell carcinoma
C. Is less likely to be associated with clubbing than squamous cell carcinoma
D. Is more likely in a non-smoker than squamous cell carcinoma
E. Is the most common type of scar carcinoma

T T F T T

Clubbing and hypertrophic pulmonary osteoarthropathy and hypercoagulability are more frequent in adenocarcinomas.

Q37 A solitary lung nodule

A. Is defined as being <3 cm in diameter
B. Most often is malignant
C. With smooth, well-defined margins is diagnostic of a benign cause
D. With diffuse solid calcification is characteristic of a malignant origin
E. Showing enhancement of less than 15 Hounsfield Units after contrast is strongly predictive of a malignancy

T F F F F

Solitary pulmonary nodules are defined as focal, round or oval areas of increased opacity in the lung that measure less than 3 cm in diameter. They are caused by a variety of disorders including neoplasms, infection, inflammation, and vascular and congenital abnormalities. Although most solitary pulmonary nodules are benign, 30%–40% are malignant. Most nodules with smooth, well-defined margins are benign, whilst a lobulated contour implies uneven growth that is associated with malignancy. It is important to note that 20-25% of tumours contravene this rule. Nodules with an irregular or spiculated margin with distortion of adjacent vessels (sunburst or corona radiate like appearance), are likely to be malignant. There are four benign patterns of calcification described: central, diffuse solid, laminated, and "popcorn like." The first three patterns are typically seen with previous infections such as histoplasmosis or tuberculosis. Popcorn like calcification is characteristic of chondroid calcification in a hamartoma. Diffuse and amorphous or punctate calcification is seen in malignancies. Nodular enhancement of less than 15 HU after contrast is strongly predictive of a benign lesion, whereas enhancement of more than 20 HU typically indicates malignancy.

Q38 Squamous cell carcinoma of the oesophagus

A. Is increasing in incidence in the western hemisphere
B. Is a complication of caustic ingestion
C. Occurs in a Zenker's diverticulum
D. Is not associated with alcohol and tobacco use as is the case with adenocarcinoma of the oesophagus
E. Is associated with human papilloma virus infection

F T T F T

Squamous cell carcinoma was the more common type of oesophageal cancer in the past, but now makes up less than 50% of oesophageal cancers in Europe and North America. Alcohol and tobacco use are known risk factors for oesophageal squamous cell carcinoma. Infection with human papilloma virus subtypes 16 and 18 has been implicated in the pathogenesis of oesophageal squamous cell carcinoma.

Q39 Which of the following describes thoracic actinomycosis correctly?

A. It is caused by filamentous fungi
B. Lesions are characterised by the presence of companion bacteria
C. It mimics features of lung cancer
D. It commonly causes constrictive pericarditis
E. It is best treated with long term penicillin

F T T F T

Thoracic actinomycosis is caused by a gram positive bacteria. Mediastinal involvement is rare. Treatment is with Penicillin for 3 months.

Q40 Which of the following are true of Kartagener's syndrome?

A. It is transmitted in an autosomal recessive manner
B. It is associated with dextrocardia
C. It is a cause of bronchiectasis
D. It is associated with infertility
E. Bronchiectasis tends to involve especially the lung apices

F T F T F

Kartagener's syndrome is a triad of situs inversus, chronic sinusitis and bronchiectasis and is associated with a more generalised condition known as immotile cilia syndrome. Males may demonstrate infertility secondary to immotile spermatozoa. Bronchiectasis tends to involve especially the lung bases.

Q41 Which of the following are true regarding the lymph node stations in lung cancer?

A. N0 is designated when regional lymph nodes cannot be assessed
B. Lymph node station 5 drains the left upper lobe
C. Metastasis to ipsilateral scalene or supraclavicular lymph nodes is designated N3 disease
D. If involvement of intrapulmonary nodes is by direct extension of the primary tumour it is designated as N0 disease
E. Metastasis to subcarinal lymph nodes is designated as N3 disease

F T T F F

NX is designated when regional lymph nodes cannot be assessed. Metastasis to contralateral mediastinal, contralateral hilar, ipsilateral or contralateral scalene, or supraclavicular lymph node is designated N3 disease. Metastasis to ipsilateral peribronchial and/or ipsilateral hilar lymph nodes, and intrapulmonary nodes including involvement by direct extension of the primary tumour is designated N1 disease. Metastasis to ipsilateral mediastinal and/or subcarinal lymph node(s) is designated as N2 disease. Reference - American Joint Committee on Cancer.: AJCC Cancer Staging Manual. 6th ed. New York, NY: Springer, 2002, pp 167-181.

Q42 Regarding drug therapy in pulmonary tuberculosis

A. Contacts of patients with active disease should receive prophylaxis with Isoniazid
B. Latent tuberculosis is treated with ethambutol
C. Multidrug resistant tuberculosis is defined as resistance to pyrazinamide
D. Rifampicin can be used during pregnancy
E. In managing patients with treatment failure a single additional drug is added to the failing regimen

T F F T F

Chemotherapy of TB consists of prevention of infection, also known as primary chemoprophylaxis, when isoniazid is given to prevent infection in contacts. In the treatment of latent tuberculosis, also known as secondary chemoprophylaxis, isoniazid is given for 6 months to prevent disease in infected persons (asymptomatic Mycobacterium tuberculosis positive individuals). Multidrug resistant tuberculosis is defined as resistance to isoniazid and rifampicin. Rifampicin, isoniazid, ethambutol, and pyrazinamide can be used during pregnancy. Streptomycin is not given due to foetal ototoxicity. In managing patients with treatment failure adding a single drug leads to acquired resistance to the new drug and hence two, or preferably three, new drugs to which susceptibility could be inferred should be added to lessen the likelihood of further acquired resistance.

Q43 Which of the following are true of aspergillomas?

A. They occur as a result of a necrotising aspergillus pneumonia
B. They occcur in preexisting lung cavities
C. They are associated with haemoptysis in 10-20% of patients
D. Aspergillus precipitin IgG antibody tests are usually positive
E. They may be treated with a trial of Itraconazole or Amphotericin-B

T T F T T

Haemoptysis occurs in 40-60% of patients. Elevated aspergillous precipitin levels are present in approximately half of the patients.

Q44 Which of the following are true regarding histoplasmosis?

A. In most people infection is asymptomatic
B. It is aquired by inhalation of bacteria from bird droppings
C. It causes a chronic cavitating lung disease
D. It is a common cause of a fibrosing mediastinitis
E. It is best treated with a long term course of penicillin

T F T T F

Histoplasmosis is aquired by inhalation of spores and best treated with a course of an antifungal such as Ketoconazole.

Q45 Which of the following statements regarding predisposing factors for oesophageal carcinoma are true?

A. Tylosis predisposes to oesophageal cancer
B. Plummer Vinson syndrome predisposes to adenocarcinoma
C. Barrett's oesophagus is associated with a two fold increase in the likelihood of oesophageal adenocarcinoma
D. The incidence is increased in hiatus hernia
E. Cigarette smoking is associated with an increased risk for squamous cell carcinoma

T F F F T

Tylosis and Plummer Vinson syndrome are associated with an increased risk of squamous cell carcinoma. Barrette's oesophagus is associated with a thirty fold increase in the likelihood of adenocarcinoma. Cigarette smoking is associated with a 10 fold increase in risk for squamous cell carcinoma, and a 2-3 fold increase in risk for adenocarcinoma.

Q46 Which of the following are true regarding adenoid cystic carcinoma of the trachea?

A. It has an insidious onset, a slow growth pattern, and shows perineural growth
B. Haemoptysis is more common than in patients with squamous cell carcinoma of the trachea
C. It tends to metastasise to regional lymph nodes
D. Haematogenous metastases to the lung are uncommon
E. The five-year survival after resection is worse than with squamous cell carcinoma of the trachea

T F F F F

Haemoptysis is more common in patients with squamous cell carcinoma, often leading to earlier diagnosis. Only about 10% of adenoid cystic carcinomas will metastasise to regional lymph nodes. Haematogenous metastases to the lung are not uncommon, described in 1/3 of patients. The five-year survival after resection is approximately 75% as compared to 50% for the squamous type.

Q47 Which are true regarding chondrosarcoma of the ribs?

A. It occurs in the fifth or sixth decades.
B. It is the most common malignant tumour of the sternum or rib
C. Its tumour cells produce a pure hyaline cartilage
D. Treatment of chondrosarcoma is with chemotherapy
E. Prognosis is related to histological grade

T T T F T

Treatment of chondrosarcoma is wide surgical excision. There is a very limited role for chemotherapy or radiation. There is an inverse relationship between histological grade and prognosis.

Q48 Which are true of bronchoalveolar cell carcinoma of the lung?

A. The cell of origin is the type I pneumocyte
B. The cells secrete mucin
C. Chemotherapy is the preferred treatment
D. It is a form of adenocarcinoma
E. It has a strong association with smoking

F T F T F

The cell of origin is the type II pneumocyte. Thus the tumour cells secrete mucin and surfactant apoprotein, which can lead to bronchorrhoea. Surgery is the preferred treatment if the tumour can be resected. It is a form of adenocarcinoma, a non-small cell carcinoma of the lung. It represents approximately 10 to 25 percent of all adenocarcinoma cases. Although it is smoking-related, its relationship with smoking is less strong than with other types of NSCLC.

Q49 Which of the following regarding Nocardia asteroids are true?

A. It is a gram positive organism
B. It is acid-fast
C. Cough is a prominent feature of infection with it
D. The typical lesions of nocardiosis are abscesses extensively infiltrated with neutrophils
E. Penicillins are the antimicrobials of choice

T T T T F

It is an aerobic, gram positive and mildly acid-fast organism that appears as beaded, branching filaments with also bacillar or coccal forms. Cough is prominent and is often productive of small quantities of thick, non-odorous, purulent sputum. Sulphonamides are the antimicrobials of choice.

Q50 Achalasia cardia of the oesophagus

A. Is characterised by loss of ganglion cells in the myenteric plexus of Auerbach
B. The lower oesophageal sphincter fails to relax
C. Occurs more often in females than males
D. Patients with achalasia with a dilated and tortuous oesophagus have a poorer outcome following oesophageal myotomy
E. Is associated with an increased risk for oesophageal cancer

T T F T T

In the early stages of achalasia, a mixed inflammatory infiltrate of T cells, mast cells, and oeosinophils is seen, in association with myenteric neural fibrosis and selective loss of inhibitory postganglionic neurons from the Auerbach plexus. Achalasia has no sex predilection. In the presence of impaired peristalsis patients with a tortuous oesophagus have restricted emptying by gravity. An increased risk for oesophageal cancer occurs, especially in patients with a long history of achalasia.

Q51 Which are true of the thoracic outlet syndrome?

A. It is most often neurogenic
B. Overall it is more often diagnosed in females
C. The ulnar nerve conduction velocity across the thoracic outlet is 72 m/sec
D. Cervical ribs are found in most patients with arterial thoracic outlet syndrome

E. Surgery is the preferred mode of management

T T F T F

Thoracic outlet syndrome is a group of disorders where compression, stretch or irritation of the neurovascular structures occurs at the thoracic outlet. The normal ulnar nerve conduction velocity across the thoracic outlet is 72 m/sec and it is reduced in the thoracic outlet syndrome. Surgery is associated with a risk of damage to local structures and incomplete resolution of symptoms and should be avoided, except for the most severe cases.

Q52 Which are correct descriptions of hypertrophic osteoarthropathy?

A. It occurs in approximately 5% of patients with bronchogenic carcinoma
B. It occurs in approximately 50% of patients with pleural mesothelioma
C. It occurs in cyanotic heart disease
D. It can be an autosomal recessive condition
E. It presents as painless swollen joints

T T T F F

Benign pleural fibromas and mesotheliomas manifest the condition. In its primary form it is an autosomal dominant condition. The condition presents as a painful condition afflicting the joints.

Q53 Benign localised fibrous tumour of the pleura

A. Is associated with smoking
B. Is associated with asbestos exposure

C. In most patients is asymptomatic
D. Is a cause of hypertrophic pulmonary osteoarthropathy
E. Manifests as hypoglycaemia

F F T T T

No association exists with smoking or asbestos exposure. Paraneoplastic manifestations include hypoglycaemia reported in approximately 5% of patients and possibly related to insulin like growth factor type 2 (IGF-2).

Q54 A patient with a mediastinal tumour has normal levels of α-foetoprotein and β-HCG. Which of the following are likely?

A. Seminoma
B. Teratoma
C. A Yolk sac tumour
D. Embryonal carcinoma
E. Thymoma

T T F F T

Yolk sac tumours are positive for both α-foetoprotein and β-HCG (in 50% of the cases, although it indicates other cell types in the tumour). Embryonal carcinoma is positive for α-foetoprotein and negative for β-HCG. Elevated serum levels of β-HCG are detected in approximately 10% of mediastinal seminomas. Levels of β-HCG exceeding 100 ng/mL are unusual, and suggest the presence of non-seminomatous elements. The serum α-foetoprotein level is always normal in pure mediastinal seminoma, and any elevation of this tumour marker indicates the presence of non-seminomatous elements. Serum lactic dehydrogenase is also elevated in the majority of patients with mediastinal seminoma. The serum tumour markers β-HCG and α-foetoprotein are usually abnormal in patients with mediastinal non-seminomatous germ cell tumours. As in mediastinal seminoma, elevation of serum lactic dehydrogenase is frequent.

Q55 Regarding interposition grafting for oesophageal reconstruction

A. Jejunal grafts are resistant to ischaemia, when compared to colonic interposition grafts
B. A jejunal graft preserves propulsive peristalsis
C. The blood supply of a short colon interposition for oesophageal reconstruction is based on the left colic artery
D. Gastric reflux is the most frequent late complication of oesophageal reconstruction with colon
E. Utilisation of the stomach entails resection of the proximal half of the lesser curvature

F T T T T

Jejunal grafts are less popular because of their high sensitivity to ischaemia, greater technical difficulty, and significantly longer time of operation. On the other hand they have the advantage that they preserve propulsive peristalsis. Colonic interposition has the advantage of relative simplicity of technique, high applicability, and low risk of ischemia. Gastric reflux is the most frequent late complication of oesophageal reconstruction with colon. Resection of the proximal half of the lesser curvature excludes lymph node spread to this area. This is recommended because it is rare to find lymph node involvement in the suprapyloric region and on the greater curvature of the stomach.

Q56 Which are true regarding granular cell tumours of the oesophagus?

A. The most common site of origin in the gastrointestinal tract is the oesophagus
B. They are most often malignant
C. The most common occurrence is in adolescence
D. They stain for S-100 protein
E. Their removal is preferably by endoscopy

T F F T F

The granular cell tumour is a solitary painless nodule that arises most commonly on the skin or the tongue. The vast majority are benign. Approximately 5% to 9% of granular cell tumours have been reported in the gastrointestinal tract, most commonly in the oesophagus. It usually presents as a benign solitary lesion. Multifocal and malignant forms are known to occur. Radiographic evaluation for the presence of metastatic disease is necessary if a malignant variant is suspected. It can occur at any age but is most common in the fourth and fifth decades. Histologically, the tumours consist of spindle or polyhedral cells and the cytoplasm contains punctated oeosinophilic granules with positive immunohistochemical staining for S-100 protein. Following initial biopsy, tumours have been followed for years endoscopically with no change in size. Whilst they may be removed endoscopically it is not advised due to the tendency to recur if incompletely excised. Hence surgical removal via a thoracotomy is often preferred.

Q57 In blunt thoracic trauma

A. Traumatic atrial septal rupture is more common than ventricular septal rupture
B. Blunt cardiac injuries are diagnosed in over 80% of patients with sternal fractures

C. Most diaphragmatic injuries detected clinically involve the left side
D. Blunt tracheal injuries require surgical repair
E. Thoracic ductal injuries are managed conservatively with chest tube drainage

F F T T T

Traumatic atrial septal rupture causing an atrial septal defect is extremely uncommon. Blunt cardiac injuries are diagnosed in fewer than 20% of patients with sternal fractures. Most diaphragmatic injuries detected clinically involve the left side, although autopsy studies suggest a roughly equal incidence for both sides. Conservative management with chest tube drainage is successful in most cases of these thoracic duct injuries.

Q58 Which of the following are true regarding superior sulcus tumours?

A. The majority histologically are squamous cell carcinomas
B. Bronchoscopy and cytology are effective in the diagnosis of the majority of cases
C. The presence of N2 disease is a poor prognostic factor
D. The classic posterior approach of resection is also known as the Paulson operation
E. The anterior transcervical technique of resection is also known as the Dartevelle procedure

T F T T T

Non-small cell lung cancer is the primary aetiology associated with radiographic abnormalities in the superior sulcus. However, only 5% of non-small cell lung cancers present as superior sulcus tumours. Due to their location, bronchoscopy and cytology are only effective in the diagnosis of 10%–20% of cases. Ultrasound or

CT guided percutaneous needle biopsy is usually sufficient to make the diagnosis. Surgery consists of a posterolateral approach, an anterior transclavicular approach, a partial sternotomy, or a combined vertebrectomy and reconstruction combined with chest wall reconstruction when the vertebral body is involved.

Q59 Which are true regarding congenital diaphragmatic hernias?

A. They show a female preponderance
B. Most foramen of Morgagni defects are right-sided
C. All Morgagni hernias should be repaired to prevent intestinal obstruction
D. Morgagni hernias are repaired via a transabdominal approach
E. Bochdalek hernias can be repaired using a transabdominal or transthoracic approach

F T T T T

They show a male preponderance. Most foramen of Morgagni defects are right-sided whilst most Bochdalek hernias are left sided.

Q60 Which of the following are true regarding oesophageal motility disorders?

A. Diffuse oesophageal spasm is characterized by >20% simultaneous contractions of the oesophagus with amplitudes exceeding 30 mmHg
B. The nutcracker oesophagus is defined by an average distal oesophageal peristaltic pressure exceeding 180 mmHg during 10 or more wet swallows
C. Scleroderma is characterised by gastro-oesophageal reflux
D. In achalasia cardia the distal oesophageal spincter is hypotonic

174

E. Hypertensive lower oesophageal sphincter is defined as a 'resting' lower oesophageal sphincter pressure exceeding 45 mmHg

T T T F T

Diffuse oesophageal spasm occurs when the propagative waves do not progress correctly. A number of segments of the oesophagus contract simultaneously, preventing the propagation of the food bolus. Nutcracker oesophagus occurs when the amplitude of the contractions exceeds 2 standard deviations from normal. The contractions proceed in an organized manner, propelling food down the oesophagus. Hence these patients often present with chest pain rather than dysphagia. In scleroderma dysmotility develops as the smooth muscle of the oesophagus is replaced by fibrous tissue, gradually leading to progressive loss of peristalsis and weakening of the LOS. Motility is preserved in the proximal striated muscle portion of the oesophagus. Achalasia is characterised by a loss of intrinsic acetylcholine-containing nerves in the oesophageal body in association with the loss of the inhibitory nerves at the lower sphincter, resulting in failure of the LOS to completely relax, thus causing relative obstruction. Hypertensive lower oesophageal sphincter is defined as an elevated lower oesophageal sphincter pressure (> 45 mm Hg) with normal peristalsis.

Q61 Which of the following are true of lung abscesses?

A. They occurs most commonly in the right lower lobe
B. Aspiration of infectious material is the most frequent aetiology
C. They occur more often in edentulous patients than in dentulous patients
D. They may be associated with clubbing of the fingers

E. Surgical resection is the management of choice if it is not possible to eliminate a carcinoma as the underlying cause

T F F T T

It is unusual for edentulous patients to develop a lung abscess because they lack a periodontal flora. Hence other more sinister causes such as lung cancer need to be sought in these patients.

Q62 Which of the following are true regarding thoracic chordomas?

A. They are rapidly growing tumours
B. They are malignant tumours
C. They arise from the remnants of the notochord
D. Thoracic chordomas account for approximately 50% of all chordomas
E. The treatment of choice is surgical excision

F T T T T

Chordomas are slowly growing tumours. They arise from remnants of the notochord, which usually persists only in the nucleus pulposus of the intervertebral discs. Presentation is as a soft tissue mass in the posterior mediastinum. Thoracic chordomas account for only 1–2% of all chordomas. The treatment of choice is surgical excision and this may involve multiple surgical procedures since they have a tendency for frequent local recurrence.

Q63 The superior vena caval syndrome

A. Is caused by aneurysms of the ascending aorta
B. Is associated with tuberculosis
C. Most often is caused by a small cell lung cancer
D. Is less pronounced if the obstruction is below the entry of the azygous vein
E. Is more frequently encountered in children than in adults

T T T F F

Since superior vena caval syndrome was first described by William Hunter in 1757, the range of underlying conditions associated with it has shifted from infective causes such as tuberculosis and syphilitic aneurysms of the ascending aorta to malignant disorders, especially in Europe and North America. The most common cause is small cell bronchogenic carcinoma, followed by squamous cell carcinoma of the lung. If the obstruction is above the entry of the azygous vein, the syndrome is less pronounced as the azygous system shunts upper body venous return back to the heart. If the obstruction is below the entry of the azygous vein, more florid symptoms and signs are seen. SVC obstruction is rare in children and the most frequent malignant cause is non-Hodgkin's lymphoma.

Q64 Which of the following statements are true of bronchogenic cysts?

A. They first start appearing in adolescence
B. They are lined by ciliated columnar epithelial cells
C. They classically show contrast enhancement on CT scanning
D. They most often are intrapulmonary
E. Surgery is the treatment of choice

F T F F T

Bronchogenic cysts appear in the third trimester of intrauterine life and are hence congenital abnormalities. They classically show absence of contrast enhancement on CT scanning and do not enhance with gadolinium on MRI. Most bronchogenic cysts are located in the mediastinum. Surgical exision is the treatment of choice both to obtain a histological diagnosis, as well as to eliminate potential complications including malignant change within them.

Q65 Regarding segmentectomy for non-small cell lung cancer

   A. For a peripheral localised non-small cell lung cancer it gives an actuarial survival rate comparable with a lobectomy
   B. It offers significantly better functional preservation compared with lobectomy
   C. It may play an useful role in treatment of metachronous lesions
   D. It may result in bronchopleural fistulae
   E. It is generally associated with a mortality of 3 %

T T T T F

For T1N0M0 lesions, the actuarial survival rate at 36 months is the same following segmentectomy or lobectomy. Segmentectomy may play an useful role in treatment of metachronous or synchronous lung cancer. Small bronchi need to be looked for in the segmentectomy margin and closed after the procedure to avoid prolonged air leaks. Segmentectomy is associated with a mortality rate of 1-1.5% unless the pulmonary function is poor or it is a redo-operation.

Q66 Regarding congenital tracheo-oesophageal fistulae

A. In the commonest type, the upper oesophageal segment ends in a blind pouch with a fistula connecting the distal oesophageal segment to the trachea
B. Antenatal ultrasound shows oligohydramnios in the majority
C. They are associated with renal anomalies
D. An H-type tracheo-oesophageal fistula may present insidiously
E. Their repair is performed via a left thoracotomy

T F T T F

Antenatal ultrasound shows polyhydramnios in the majority. They are associated with two groups of anomalies. The VACTERL (Vertebral, Anal, Cardiac, Tracheal, 'Esophagus', Renal and Limb) association of congenital heart disease, intestinal atresia, imperforate anus, skeletal anomalies and renal anomalies and the CHARGE association of Coloboma, congenital Heart disease, choanal Atresia, growth and mental Retardation, Genital hypoplasia, Ear anomalies. Repair is via a right thoracotomy with the head of table elevated to avoid gastric reflux. A posterolateral thoracotomy is made through the fourth intercostal space, and a retropleural exposure is obtained with the azygous vein divided and the vagus nerve is identified.

Q67 Which of the following are true of bronchoplastic procedures?

A. Bronchoplastic resections are the treatment of choice for central carcinoid tumours
B. Bronchoplastic techniques can be used to repair traumatic airway injuries
C. Pleural coverage of the anastomosis is effective in preventing major complications due to dehiscence of the bronchial anastomosis

D. Sleeve pneumonectomies are associated with poor survival

E. The presence of N2 disease significantly worsens prognosis

T T F T T

With central carcinoid tumours bronchoplastic procedures help conserve lung tissue in relatively young patients who are active. Bronchoplastic techniques can be used to repair traumatic airway injuries and also benign airway strictures. Pleural coverage of the anastomosis has been shown to not be effective in preventing major complications due to dehiscence of the bronchial anastomosis. A pedicled muscle flap could be a valuable alternative. Bronchoplastic procedures involving sleeve pneumonectomies are associated with poor survival. Sleeve resection is an adequate operation for patients with resectable lung cancer and N0 or N1 status. The presence of N2 disease significantly worsens the prognosis and may contraindicate the use of the procedure.

Q68 Which of the following are correct regarding the chest radiographic staging of sarcoidosis?

A. A normal chest x-ray is stage 0 disease

B. Isolated hilar lymphadenopathy is stage 1 disease

C. Presence of both hilar adenopathy and pulmonary infiltrates is stage 2 disease

D. Isolated pulmonary infiltrates is stage 4 disease

E. Pulmonary fibrosis is stage 5 disease

T T T T T

Below is an outline of the chest radiographic staging of sarcoidosis.

Stage	Description
0	Normal radiograph
I	Bilateral hilar adenopathy
II	Bilateral hilar adenopathy & lung opacities
III	Lung opacities alone
IV	Parenchymal fibrosis

Q69 Which of the following are true of small cell lung cancer?

A. Risk factors for small cell lung cancer include being exposed to asbestos
B. It has a greater tendency to be widely disseminated by the time of diagnosis
C. A patient with ipsilateral supraclavicular lymph nodes is designated as having limited-stage disease
D. Has a lower likelihood of being responsive to chemotherapy and irradiation than non-small cell lung cancer
E. Absence of chromogranin A staining helps differentiate it from carcinoid

T T T F T

Risk factors for small cell lung cancer include being exposed to asbestos or radon. Compared with non-small cell lung cancer, small cell carcinoma has a greater tendency to be widely disseminated by the time of diagnosis but is much more responsive to chemotherapy and irradiation. At diagnosis, approximately 30% of patients with small cell carcinoma have tumour confined to the hemithorax of origin, the mediastinum, or the supraclavicular lymph nodes and are designated as having limited-stage disease.

Q70 Which statements are correct regarding empyema necessitans?

A. It involves soft-tissue extension of empyema
B. It may present as sinuses through the intercostal spaces on the chest wall
C. Aerobic organisms are the predominant pathogens recovered in a majority of cases
D. CT is insensitive for identifying focal pleural or chest wall abnormalities
E. Treatment of empyema necessitans involves closed or open drainage of the pleural space

T T F F T

Empyema necessitans is a soft-tissue extension of empyema leading to chest wall infection and external drainage. Anaerobic organisms are the predominant pathogens recovered in the majority of cases. Treatment of empyema necessitans involves closed or open drainage of the pleural space to prevent fibrosis and to facilitate expansion of the lung. Appropriate antibiotic therapy is also an important part of treatment. CT is a sensitive modality for differentiating pleural fluid from pleural thickening and for identifying focal pleural or chest wall abnormalities.

Q71 Hydatid cysts

A. Are caused by infection with E. multilocularis
B. Most commonly affect the lungs
C. Are characterised by an oeosinophilia
D. Are associated with positive anti-Echinococcal IgG antibodies
E. Are treated with Albendazole

F F F T T

Infection with E. multilocularis results in dense parasitic tumours in the liver, lungs, brain, and other organs, whilst it is infection with E. granulosus that typically results in the formation of cysts. Hydatid cysts most commonly affect the liver with the lungs being the second most common organ to be affected. Oeosinophilia is absent in most patients. Approximately 10% of patients with hepatic cysts and 40% with pulmonary cysts may exhibit false-negative results, especially if they are calcified. Although both are effective, albendazole is the drug of choice as its systemic absorption and penetration into cysts is superior to that of mebendazole.

Q72 Which of the following are correct regarding tuberculosis?

A. People with latent tuberculosis are infective to others
B. Multidrug-resistance is defined as TB bacilli resistant to at least isoniazid and ethambutol
C. It accounts for about 13% of AIDS deaths worldwide
D. Active respiratory tuberculosis is treated with rifampicin and isoniazid for 6 months supplemented in the first two months with pyrazinamide and ethambutol
E. Patients with active pericardial tuberculosis should be offered prednisolone 60mg/day in addition to anti-tuberculous treatment

F F T T T

Multidrug-resistant TB is defined as disease caused by TB bacilli resistant to at least isoniazid and rifampicin, the two most powerful anti-TB drugs. Pericardial disease warrants the addition of a steroid for 2-3 weeks prior to tapering it. As the guidelines for treatment can vary over time updates should be obtained from the NICE (UK) or the CDC (North America).

Q73 Which of the following are laboratory features consistent with an empyema thoracis?

    A. Protein >3g/dl
    B. pH <7.20
    C. Glucose level <50 mg/dL
    D. Lactate dehydrogenase (LDH) level >1000 IU/L
    E. Bacteria on Gram staining

T T T T T

The presence of bacteria results in metabolism and the consumption of glucose as well as the production of products of metabolism with a resultant drop in the pH. The inflammation results in a high protein content and LDH as compared to a transudate.

Q74 Which of the following are correct regarding hiatal herniae?

    A. In a sliding hiatal hernia, the lower oesophageal sphincter lies in the chest
    B. Para-oesophageal hernia are rare in children
    C. Shortness of breath is a common complaint of patients who present with sliding hernias
    D. Incarceration and strangulation are more likely with a para-oesophageal hernia
    E. Para-oesophageal hernia are managed conservatively with the use of antacids

T T F T F

The three main types of hiatal hernia are sliding, para-oesophageal, and mixed. Shortness of breath is a common complaint of patients who present with para-oesophageal hernias as the hernia enlarges due to decreased thoracic capacity. Medical management for para-oesophageal hernia is surgical correction to avoid life-threatening complications.

Q75 In tracheostomy

A. There is an increased risk of aspiration
B. Pneumothorax and pneumomediastinum following tracheostomy is more common in children
C. Tracheo-oesophageal fistula occurring as a complication should be managed conservatively
D. The most frequent site of tracheo-innominate artery fistula formation is at the distal end of the tracheostomy tube
E. Suspicion of a tracheo-innominate artery fistula should be confirmed by angiography

T T F T F

A tracheostomy can fix the trachea inhibiting its vertical excursion and preventing supraglottic closure, increasing the risk of aspiration. The higher incidence of intrathoracic complications in children is attributed to operative injury of the apical pleura because of its high position. There is no evidence that tracheo-oesophageal fistulae close spontaneously and there is an almost total mortality rate in those not operated. Surgical management is with direct closure and muscle flap interposition, or oesophageal diversion. The likelihood of a tracheo-innominate artery fistula formation is increased by low placement of the tracheotomy as well as by the presence of a high innominate artery. Suspicion of a tracheo-innominate artery fistula should be followed by removal of the tracheostomy tube and bronchoscopy with caution.

Angiography is not helpful and is likely to delay definitive treatment.

Q76 Which of the following are correct regarding mesothelioma?

A. The level of soluble mesothelin-related protein is elevated in the serum of about 75% of patients at diagnosis
B. It is associated with smoking
C. The MS01 trial is a randomized Phase III study comparing active symptom control with or without chemotherapy
D. The MesoVATS trial is a randomized Phase III study comparing surgical pleurectomy and palliative talc pleurodesis in preventing fluid recurrence
E. The MARS study is a randomized trial assessing the role of radical extrapleural pneumonectomy in early stage mesothelioma

T F T T T

The MARS (Mesothelioma And Radical Surgery) study, is a randomized trial in which one group of participants would receive chemotherapy, then extra-pleural pneomonectomy (EPP), then radiotherapy. The second group of patients would receive other types of aggressive therapy, but would not receive EPP.

Q77 Which of the following are true of pancoast tumours?

A. They rarely cause symptoms that are typically related to the lungs.
B. They may present as Horner's syndrome
C. MRI is superior to CT scanning in the evaluation of mediastinal node involvement

D. The 5-year survival rate after surgery is approximately 15%
E. Involvement of mediastinal lymph nodes reduces the median expected survival to less than 9 months

T T F F T

Horner's syndrome is characterised by ptosis, anhydrosis, enophthalmos, and meiosis. CT scan findings are much better than MRI for assessing the mediastinum to determine if the tumour has involved the mediastinal lymph nodes. The 5-year survival rate after surgery is approximately 30%.

Q78 Which of the following are correct descriptions of pleural fibromas?

A. They are aetiologically related to asbestos exposure
B. They occur as synchronous lesions
C. They are commonly associated with pleural effusions
D. They do not enhance on contrast-enhanced CT scans due to their fibrous nature
E. Surgical excision is the treatment of choice

F F F F T

No proven association exists with smoking or asbestos exposure. Synchronous lesions are extremely rare. They enhance on contrast-enhanced CT scans due to their rich vascularity.

Q79 Branchial cleft cysts are correctly described as

A. Being the most common congenital cause of a neck mass
B. Occurring due to failure of obliteration of the second branchial cleft

C. Occurring along the lower one third of the anterior border of the sternocleidomastoid muscle
D. Being bilateral in about 20-30% of the cases
E. Being endothelial cysts

T F F F T

Branchial cleft cysts are congenital cysts that arise in the lateral aspect of the neck, most often when the second branchial cleft fails to close during embryonic development. First branchial cleft cysts (10%) present in the periauricular area, second branchial cleft cysts (80-90%) can present anywhere along the anterior border of the sternocleidomastoid muscle and third and fourth branchial cleft cysts are very rare but also present along the sternocleidomastoid muscle. Branchial cleft cysts are bilateral in about 2-3% of the cases. Most cysts are epithelial lined with stratified squamous epithelium whilst a small number are lined with respiratory (ciliated columnar) epithelium.

Q80 Which are true of superior vena caval obstruction?

A. Bronchogenic small-cell carcinomas account for the majority of cases
B. In children the most important cause is a thymoma
C. Dyspnoea is often the presenting symptom
D. When due to thrombus around a central venous catheter may be treated with thrombolysis
E. Dexamethasone may be useful in acute situations

T F T T T

The most common cause is lymph node metastases from primary bronchial small cell carcinoma. In children the most important causes are T cell leukaemia and lymphoma.

Q81 With endoscopic ultrasound of the oesophagus

A. The oesophageal wall is delineated as a 3 layered structure
B. Discrimination of Stages T1 and T2 from T3 and T4 is highly effective.
C. N (lymph node) staging has a lower performance than that of T (tumour) staging
D. Staging for metastases is highly satisfactory
E. Endoscopic ultrasound does not provide an accurate assessment of coeliac axis lymphadenopathy

F T T F F

The endoscopic ultrasound (7.5-12 MegaHz) is able to delineate the oesophageal wall as a 5 layered structure. The histological correlates of the EUS image of the oesophagus are: first layer (hyperechoic) - superficial mucosa; second layer (hypoechoic) - deep mucosa; third layer (hyperechoic) - submucosa; fourth layer (hypoechoic) - muscularis propria; fifth layer (hyperechoic) - adventitia. Ability to visualise the oesophagus in this detail provides accurate T staging of oesophageal cancer, i.e. the degree of tumour infiltration into the wall layers. Staging for metastases using endoscopic ultrasound alone is not satisfactory. CT and positron emission tomography are used to detect distant metastases. Endoscopic ultrasound provides an accurate assessment of coeliac axis lymphadenopathy (local M stage), the presence of which represents distant metastasis and is associated with a worse prognosis.

Q82 Which of the following are correct regarding pectus excavatum?

A. It is the most common type of congenital chest wall deformity
B. It is associated with scoliosis
C. It is associated with a family history in a third of patients

D. It is associated with Marfan syndrome in a third of patients
E. The Nuss procedure involves excision and turning over of the sternum

T T T F F

Pectus excavatum (also known as funnel chest or trichterbrust), is responsible for approximately 90% of congenital disorders of the chest wall. Approximately 15% of patients have scoliosis. Approximately 2% of patients have Marfan syndrome and the defect tends to be more severe in them (Shamberger, 1988). The Nuss procedure involves inserting a custom bent curved metal bar underneath the sternum through lateral chest incisions. The bar is then flipped over such that the convexity is upwards. The bar is then secured to the lateral aspect of the chest wall and/or ribs and left in place for 2-3 years.

Q83 Features of a VATS sympathetectomy are correctly described in which of the following statements?

A. The sympathetic chain is divided above the stellate ganglion (T1)
B. The division of the accessory fibres of Kuntz is achieved by extending the dissection medial to the sympathetic chain
C. Severe compensatory sweating may occur as a result of the procedure
D. Oxygen saturation monitoring by a pulse oxymeter is a reliable method to detect an increase in circulation after sympathectomy
E. It is not effective in the treatment of patients with Raynaud's phenomenon

F F T T F

Two points of agreement on VATS sympathectomy found in the literature are that the sympathetic chain should be interrupted below the stellate ganglion (T1) since the division or thermal injury of the upper two thirds of T1 may cause an ipsilateral Horner's syndrome, and that the sympathectomy should include the sympathetic fibres described by Kuntz, usually found laterally to the sympathetic chain, which represent an aberrant accessory pathway of nerve conduction. The division of the accessory fibres of Kuntz is achieved by extending the dissection laterally onto the rib for 3–5 cm. Some authors describe clipping, without division, of the chain as a method to provide symptom control which can be reversed should severe compensatory sweating occur. Recently, the use of the ultrasonic scalpel to divide the chain has been advocated in view of a reduced likelihood of Horner's syndrome. Other than palmar hyperhydrosis and facial flushing it has been successfully used to treat Raynaud's phenomenon and reflex sympathetic dystrophy.

Q84 Which of the following are correct statements on pneumothorax?

A. The recurrence rate for a spontaneous pneumothorax is around 40%
B. The mortality rate associated with secondary pneumothorax is around 5%
C. Smoking increases the risk for spontaneous pneumothorax
D. Pneumothoraces <20% may be followed with serial x-rays
E. Surgical management with a thoracoscopic approach is associated with recurrence rates of 2-5%

T F T T T

The recurrence rate for both primary and secondary spontaneous pneumothorax is about 40%. The mortality rate associated with secondary pneumothorax is high at around 15%.

Q85 Which of the following descriptions regarding tumours of the diaphragm are correct?

A. They are predominantly benign lesions
B. Lipoma is the most common benign tumour of the diaphragm
C. Neurogenic tumours of the diaphragm are associated with hypertrophic pulmonary arthropathy
D. The most common primary malignant lesion is a leiomyosarcoma
E. Blood borne metastatic implants are rare with tumours of the diaphragm

F T T F T

Malignant neoplasms of the diaphragm predominate over benign lesions. Approximately half of neurogenic tumours of the diaphragm are associated with hypertrophic pulmonary arthropathy. The majority of primary malignant tumours found in the diaphragm are of fibrous tissue origin (fibrosarcoma, fibroangioendothelioma) or undifferentiated sarcomas. Other less common malignant tumours include mixed cell sarcoma, rhabdomyosarcoma, neurofibrosarcoma, haemangioendothelioma, haemangiopericytoma, and leiomyosarcoma. Metasatic disease is usually due to direct invasion from adjacent thoracic and abdominal structures.

Q86 Regarding foreign bodies of the airway

A. Most airway foreign body aspirations occur in young children
B. They most commonly are due to metallic foreign bodies
C. In adults, bronchial foreign bodies tend to be lodged in the right main bronchus rather than the left main bronchus
D. Bleeding is the most common complication

E. Antibiotics need to be prescribed after removal of the foreign body

T F T F F

Most airway foreign body aspirations occur in children aged 1-3 years. They most commonly are due to vegetable matter such as peanuts. The incidence of metallic foreign body aspirations, is less frequent. In adults, bronchial foreign bodies tend to be lodged in the right main bronchus because of its lesser angle of deviation from the long axis of the trachea than the left bronchus and also because of the location of the carina to the left of the midline. Pneumonia and atelectasis are the most common complications that occur. Antibiotics usually do not need to be prescribed because the source of infection has been removed.

Q87 Which following statements are correct regarding thoracoplasty?

A. It is used to treat chronic thoracic empyema
B. It is used in the management of bronchopleural fistula
C. It is contraindicated bilaterally
D. It may result in an impaired cough mechanism
E. It results in kyphosis in the majority of patients

T T F T F

Thoracoplasty has been used in the treatment of bilateral tuberculous empyema. The cough mechanism may be impaired by the area of unsupported chest wall. It has been found in studies that scoliosis develops in over 99 per cent of cases. The angle of curvature correlates closely with the number of ribs removed. If the head, neck and tubercle of the rib and the transverse process of the corresponding vertebra are all removed the degree of scoliosis is increased.

Q88 Which of the following regarding blunt injury to the diaphragm are correct?

A. The majority of blunt diaphragmatic ruptures result from motor vehicle accidents
B. The majority of blunt diaphragmatic ruptures occur on the left side
C. Bilateral rupture occurs in 25% of patients
D. Diaphragmatic rupture is associated with thoracic aortic disruption in approximately 10% of patients
E. Chest radiography is the single most important diagnostic study

T T F T T

The majority (over 80%), of blunt diaphragmatic ruptures occur on the left side. Right-sided ruptures are associated with more severe injuries. They require greater force of impact, and it is possible that the liver provides protection. Bilateral rupture occurs in less than 10% of cases. Diaphragmatic rupture and thoracic aortic disruption are both associated in blunt trauma and important to consider. Chest radiography is the single most important diagnostic study and may show elevation of the hemidiaphragm, a bowel pattern in the chest, or a nasogastric tube curling back up into the chest. The initial chest radiograph is non-diagnostic in around a third of patients and a repeat may be helpful. The findings may be masked in intubated patients who are being positive-pressure ventilated.

Q89 In large bullous disease of the lung

A. Most patients with bullae have a significant history of cigarette smoking
B. It causes an obstructive lung pathophysiology
C. Large bullae are associated with a risk of cancer that is higher than in normal lung parenchyma
D. An asymptomatic bulla occupying 20% of the hemithorax is an indication for surgical resection
E. Postoperative air leaks should be managed conservatively

T F T F T

Although the background lung disease may be obstructive in nature, a large bulla will cause a restrictive pathophysiology by compressing adjacent normal lung. Bullae should always be completely resected since the risk of cancer is over 30 times higher than in the normal lung parenchyma. An asymptomatic bulla occupying 30% or greater of the hemithorax or symptoms due to complications such as infection are considered indications for surgical resection. Postoperative air leaks should be managed conservatively as they relate to the diseased lung tissue along the staple margins and will usually stop with time.

Q90 Which statements are true of oesophageal perforation?

A. It occurs most frequently after instrumentation
B. The interval between perforation and treatment is a prognostic factor
C. Surgical emphysema in the neck is an uncommon sign in oesophageal perforation
D. Perforations of the intra-thoracic oesophagus are treated conservatively

E. Late retropharyngeal abscess is described in up to 20% of patients with conservatively treated cervical perforations

T T F F T

Oesophageal perforations occur most frequently after instrumentation with external trauma accounting for fewer than 10% of cases, the majority of which are penetrating injuries from stab and gunshot wounds. Oesophageal injury from blunt trauma is rare. An interval longer than 36h between perforation and treatment is associated with an approximately 50% mortality. In a retrospective review by Triggiani and Belsey (Thorax 1977) the most important diagnostic sign was surgical emphysema in the neck. Perforations of the intrathoracic oesophagus, require emergency resuscitation and immediate thoracotomy. Perforations of the cervical oesophagus may be treated conservatively.

Q91 Which are true regarding mediastinal germ cell tumours?

A. They are histologically identical to their gonadal counterparts
B. Mature teratomas occur with approximately equal frequency in male and female subjects
C. Teratomas are the most common mediastinal germ cell tumours
D. Approximately 10% of patients with pure seminoma have an elevated α-foetoprotein level
E. Non-seminomatous malignant germ cell tumours are uniquely associated with haematological malignancies

T T T F T

Mediastinal germ cell tumours (teratomas, seminomas, and non-seminomatous malignant germ cell tumours) are a heterogeneous group of benign and malignant neoplasms thought to originate from primitive germ cells "misplaced" in the mediastinum during early embryogenesis. Mature teratoma represents approximately 60-70% of mediastinal germ cell tumours. Approximately 10% of patients with pure seminoma may have an elevated β-HCG level, but not an elevated α-foetoprotein level. Non-seminomatous malignant germ cell tumours are uniquely associated with haematologic malignancies and approximately 20% of patients have Klinefelter's syndrome.

Q92 Indications for rigid bronchoscopy over flexible bronchoscopy are

A. Massive haemoptysis
B. Foreign body removal
C. Transbronchial biopsy for interstitial lung disease
D. Laser resection of obstructive malignant lesions
E. Suspected extrinsic allergic alveolitis

T T F T F

The rigid bronchoscope with a distal side port allows ventilation of the contralateral lung while working within an ipsilateral main bronchus. It also allows the insertion of a wide suction tube for suctioning out blood clot and tissue debris. In addition grasping forceps may be used for retrieval of foreign bodies. Transbronchial biopsy for interstitial disease and bronchoalveolar lavage for suspected extrinsic allergic alveolitis is easily performed by flexible bronchoscopy.

Q93 In assessment of operative risk in patients undergoing lung resection

A. A low predicted postoperative FEV1 is a strong indicator of outcome from surgery
B. Age is a major risk factor when adjusted for other co-morbid conditions
C. Age is a greater risk factor for pneumonectomy than for a lobectomy
D. Walking patients up one or two flights is an adequate stress to predict tolerance of surgery
E. Smoking cessation before surgery can reduce the risk of surgery

T F T F T

A low predicted postoperative FEV1 appears to be the best indicator of patients at high risk for complications, and it was the only significant correlate of complications when the effect of other potential risk factors was controlled for in a multivariate analysis (Kearney and colleagues 1994). Age is a minor risk factor when adjusted for other co-morbid conditions, especially if the functional status is 0 with no co-morbidity. Pollock et al. Chest 1993 found linear increases in VO2 with stair climbing. In order to reach a VO2 of 20ml/kg/min, subjects had to walk 4.6 flights of stairs, suggesting that walking patients up one or two flights is an inadequate screen. Smoking cessation even for a short period of 2 months before surgery has been shown to reduce the risk of surgery.

Q94 Which of the following are true regarding interstitial lung disease?

A. A ground glass appearance on a HRCT scan section suggests a fibrotic reaction

B. Transbronchial biopsy provides a diagnosis in the majority of patients with sarcoidosis

C. Vasculitis or collagen vascular diseases are more likely the cause in younger individuals

D. Diffusing capacity for carbon monoxide (DLCO) is generally reduced

E. It is a cause of isolated right sided heart failure

F T T T T

On a HRCT scan "ground glass" appearance is equated histologically with a cellular reaction, whereas a "reticular nodular" appearance is likely to reflect more advanced, less cellular, fibrotic areas. Transbronchial biopsy during fiberoptic bronchoscopy provides relatively small samples of tissue resulting in a confident pathologic diagnosis in only a minority of patients, due to the patchy distribution of the majority of these diseases. An exception is sarcoidosis, where the yield can be significantly higher. It is a cause of isolated right sided heart failure (cor pulmonale).

Q95 In Fibrothorax

A. The chest radiograph shows crowding of ipsilateral ribs

B. Computed tomography (CT) of the chest is the imaging modality of choice

C. Malignancy must be included in the differential diagnosis

D. Decortication entails peeling off of the visceral pleura

E. Drug therapy is the treatment of choice for tuberculous empyema

T T T F T

The chest radiograph shows crowding of ipsilateral ribs. CT of the chest is the imaging modality of choice for delineating abnormalities of the pleural space and defining the character of the pleural disease process. CT scanning can assess the extent and thickness of pleural involvement and characterise associated parenchymal disease such as fibrosis, bronchiectasis, and malignancy. Malignancy must be included in the differential diagnosis of fibrothorax and ruled out. During decortication the fibrous rind is peeled off the visceral pleura as best possible. Drug therapy is the treatment of choice for tuberculous empyema. Decortication may also be performed to treat pleural effusions that persist despite long-term medical therapy.

Q96 Which of the following are correct regarding oesophageal duplication cysts?

A. The majority of oesophageal cysts occur in the lower third of the oesophagus
B. Dysphagia is the most common symptom
C. The majority of cysts are diagnosed in adults
D. They usually communicate with the lumen of the oesophagus
E. They should always be resected

T T F F T

Sixty percent of oesophageal cysts occur in the lower third of the oesophagus, whilst the remainder are approximately equally distributed between the proximal and middle third. Difficulty swallowing from compression is the most common symptom. Furthermore cysts in the upper third of the oesophagus can cause respiratory symptoms from compression of the tracheobronchial tree, and those in the middle third can cause retrosternal discomfort. The majority of cysts are diagnosed during childhood. They do not usually communicate with the lumen of the oesophagus. All cysts should be resected when possible as, although rare, malignant degeneration can occur.

Q97 Benign oesophageal strictures are correctly described as

A. Accounting for 70-80% of all cases of oesophageal strictures
B. Being associated with an increased risk of pulmonary aspiration
C. Being associated with rapidly progressive dysphagia for solids as the most common presenting symptom
D. Being a contraindication to dilatation due to the risk of rupture
E. Being associated with a third of patients requiring repeat dilation in 1 year despite optimal acid suppression

T T F F T

Peptic strictures are the effect of gastro-oesophageal reflux induced oesophagitis, and usually originate from the squamo-columnar junction. Gradually progressive dysphagia for solids is the most common presenting symptom and rapid progression should raise the possibility of a malignant cause. Dilatation may be required for symptom relief. Progressive dilation of peptic strictures gives effective relief of dysphagia in the majority of cases, with a low rate of complications. The recurrence rate doubles if no acid suppression is used.

Q98 Which of the following are true of malignant pleural effusions?

A. They are most often caused by breast cancer in female patients
B. They are excluded if fluid analysis shows a transudate
C. Due to non-small cell lung cancer are likely to respond to systemic chemotherapy
D. They are more suitably treated with pleurectomy than with pleurodesis
E. They are best treated with insertion of a pleuro-peritoneal shunt

T F F F F

In female patients, about 40% of malignant effusions are caused by breast cancer. Malignancy usually causes an exudative effusion but can cause a transudative effusion occasionally by lymphatic blockade. Malignant effusions due to chemotherapy-resistant tumours, like non-small cell lung cancer, are not likely to respond to systemic therapy. Pleurectomy is effective in controlling malignant pleural effusions, but the morbidity is severe and pleurodesis is hence often preferred. Insertion of a pleuro-peritoneal shunt is likely to disseminate the malignancy to the peritoneum if this is disease free and whilst improving dyspnoea is not the preferred treatment in the majority of patients.

Q99 In patients with malignant mesothelioma treated with aggressive surgical approaches, factors associated with improved long-term survival include

A. Male gender
B. Epithelial histology
C. Negative lymph nodes
D. Negative surgical margins

E. Absence of a history of exposure to asbestos

F T T T F

Important prognostic factors in patients with malignant mesothelioma are stage, age, performance status, and histology. From amongst them for those patients treated with aggressive surgical approaches, nodal status, histology and resection margins are important prognostic factors.

Q100 Which statements are true of solitary lung nodules?

A. They are defined as less than 3 cm in diameter
B. They are typically asymptomatic
C. They are most often benign
D. They are less likely to be malignant in male patients than in female patients
E. They are caused by Dirofilaria immitis

T T T F T

Sixty percent of all solitary lung nodules are benign. In areas where there are infectious agents (especially fungi) that cause solitary lung nodules, the percentage of benign lesions increases. Factors increasing the chances of malignancy include a history of cigarette smoking, age >45 years, male gender, respiratory symptoms and a history of cancer elsewhere. Factors that increase the chance that the nodule is benign include the patient coming from an area with a high incidence of histoplasmosis or coccidomycosis. Dirofilaria immitis is a rare parasitic infestation seen in pet owners/people working with animals, and is caused by a type of filarial worm. Adults are parasites mainly of the chambers of the right side of the heart and pulmonary artery. Microfilariae can be carried through to the lungs.

CHAPTER 4

Single Best Answer Questions

Each question is followed by five answers. Please select the single best response to each.

1) In the treatment of patients with coronary artery disease

   A. Patients with left main stem disease are best treated with PCI

   B. Patients with three vessel disease have best long term outcome when treated with PCI

   C. Patients with impaired LV systolic function have a prognostic advantage when treated with PCI rather than surgery

   D. There is evidence from randomised controlled studies for the prognostic benefit of coronary artery surgery in patients with severe coronary artery disease

   E. Patients with impaired LV function should not be offered cardiac surgery because they have little to gain from an operation

2) Analysis of cardiac surgical databases has shown that cardiac surgical mortality is influenced by

   A. The presence of mild mitral regurgitation

   B. The number of coronary grafts that are required

C. The patient being hypercholesterolaemic
D. The gender of the patient
E. The presence or absence of diabetes mellitus

3) Regarding the performance of conduits used for coronary artery bypass grafting

A. 10% of saphenous vein grafts are occluded within one month
B. The average length of life of a saphenous vein graft is 25 years
C. Lipid lowering therapy can prolong the life of saphenous vein grafts beyond 25 years
D. Saphenous vein grafts last longer than arterial grafts
E. The most commonly used arterial graft is the radial artery

4) Regarding surgery for pneumothorax

A. It should always be offered only after a recurrent episode
B. It should also be performed on the contralateral side prophylactically
C. Pneumothorax is treated often by surgical talc pleurodesis
D. It is usually unsuccessful in patients with Marfan's syndrome
E. A bullectomy complimented with a pleurectomy has a lower recurrence than an isolated bullectomy

5) The treatment of heart failure is most accurately described by which of the following statements?

A. The incidence of heart failure after an acute myocardial infarction is not influenced by PCI

B. Dysrythmias are the most common cause of death for patients hospitalised with an acute myocardial infarction

C. Ventricular remodelling surgery attempts to restore the geometry of the left ventricle

D. Bi-ventricular pacing is a contraindication for surgical left ventricular remodelling

E. Ventricular support devices have no role in the management of heart failure

6) Which of the following statements best describes sternal wound breakdown after cardiac surgery?

A. The presence of superficial tissue healing excludes the presence of sternal dehiscence

B. When associated with deep sternal wound infection requires a temperature $>38°$ C to make the diagnosis

C. It is always related to infection

D. It has no correlation to the BMI in female patients

E. The CRP is a good guide to the response to antibiotics

7) Which of the following are true regarding statins?

A. They lower the level of cholesterol in the blood by increasing breakdown of cholesterol by the liver.

B. They slow the formation of new atherosclerotic plaques

C. When taken with verapamil, the likelihood of myopathy is occasionally increased

D. They are very effective in lowering HDL cholesterol

E. They reduce the likelihood of coronary disease in all populations

8) Regarding the management of patients with coronary artery disease found to have significant carotid artery disease

A. The stroke risk is least when the CEA is performed before CABG
B. The stroke risk is least when the CEA and CABG are performed concurrently
C. The stroke risk is least when CABG is performed before CEA
D. The stroke risk for CABG is not influenced by the presence of carotid disease
E. CABG should not be performed in patients with carotid disease

Answers to questions

1. D
2. D
3. A
4. E
5. C
6. E
7. B
8. A

CHAPTER 5

Sample EMI Questions

Questions 1 - 4

The figure below shows left ventricular Pressure–Time curve responses 'a' to 'g' in a 59 year old patient admitted with unstable angina under the cardiologist. Curve 'b' represents the trace when his angina subsequently settled that evening after medical therapy.

Select the best response from them for Questions 1-4. Each response may be used more than once

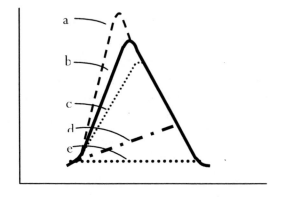

Pressure

a

b

c

d

e

Time

Question 1

The next morning the patient's spouse visited. During the visit a heated argument ensured and the patient complained of a recurrence in chest pain. The blood pressure was 90/60 mmHg. The pain was not relieved by medication and an acute coronary syndrome was diagnosed. Which left ventricular Pressure–Time curve would be likely obtained immediately after the diagnosis of the acute coronary syndrome?

Question 2

The patient went onto have coronary artery bypass grafting with cold blood cardioplegia for myocardial preservation. Which left ventricular Pressure–Time curve would be likely obtained soon after release of the aortic cross clamp subsequent to coronary artery bypass grafting?

Question 3

On transfer to the intensive care unit postoperatively the systemic pressure was noted to be dropping despite an adequate central venous pressure and the patient was commenced on a low dose adrenaline infusion. A very good response was noted. Which left ventricular Pressure–Time curve would be likely to have been obtained after commencing an infusion of adrenaline on the intensive care unit?

Question 4

The patient recovered well from the operation to be subsequently discharged home a week after surgery. Which left ventricular Pressure–Time curve would be likely obtained on discharge home?

Questions 5 - 7

Please select the best response from amongst the following for questions 5 to 7. Each stem may be used more than once as the suitable response.

a) A β-haemolytic streptococus
b) An α-haemolytic streptococus
c) Carcinoid mitral valve disease
d) Aortic stenosis due to a bicuspid valve
e) Aortic regurgitation
f) Ascending aortic replacement
g) Heart-lung transplantation
i) Dissection of the aorta
j) Transection of the aorta
k) A myocardial infarction

Question 5

A 28 year old pregnant female presents with excessive shortness of breath to your practice. On auscultation she is in heart failure and you here a diastolic murmur in the mitral area. In her past medical history she suffered from an episode of sore throat and arthralgia when 11 years of age. She was living in South America at the time and arrived in this country when she was 21 years of age. You refer the patient immediately to the on call cardiology team, who perform an echocardiogram. What is the likely cause of her childhood sore throat?

Question 6

The next day you see a patient who 5 years previously presented to you as an emergency and had an emergency heart operation. He brings his

21 year old basket-baller son who has been complaining of severe and worsening pain between the scapular blades for approximately an hour. What operation do you think the father had previously?

Question 7

Over the weekend your colleague surgeon on take is called to the hospitals major trauma room to see a young driver of a car that had crashed into a road side tree at high speed. The patient was not known to have any past medical problems and had appeared comfortable. A chest radiograph had shown a slight widening of his superior mediastinum. The patient was investigated further and subsequently had emergency surgery. What is the likely diagnosis that led to the emergency surgery?

Answers to questions 1 - 4

Q 1 – c
Q 2 – d
Q 3 – a
Q4 – b

Answers to questions 5 - 7

Q 5 – a
Q 6 – f
Q 7 – j

ISBN 142515814-5

9 781425 158149